Ayurveda Revolutionized

Integrating Ancient and Modern Ayurveda

Edward F. Tarabilda

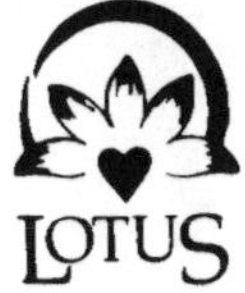

DISCLAIMER

This book is a reference work. It is not intended to be used for treatment, diagnosis or to prescribe. The information contained herein should in no way be considered a substitute for consultation with a duly-licensed health-care professional.

Cover art, design and page layout: Paul Bond, Art & Soul Design
Editor: Parvati Markus

First Edition 1997

Printed in the United States of America

Library of Congress Cataloging-in-Publication-Data
Ayurveda Revolutionized, Integrating Ancient and Modern Ayurveda
includes bibliographical references.
ISBN 0-914955-38-1 97-71503
CIP

Published by:
Lotus Press, P.O. Box 325, Twin Lakes, Wisconsin 53181

ACKNOWLEDGMENTS

Thanks to Lenny Blank for his invaluable suggestions in improving the overall presentation, writing the Preface, and for producing this book for Lotus Press.

My deep appreciation to David Frawley for providing the Foreword to the book.

I also wish to thank Bernadette Cardinale, a teacher of the "Art of Multi-Dimensional Living," for her devoted friendship, creative imput and finishing touch edit of this book.

I want to express thanks to Parvati Markus for her skillful editing.

Lastly, I thank and acknowledge Santosh Krinsky for seeing the great potential of this ancient paradigm of healing, even as far back as the late 1980's, and encouraging me to make it available for the health and well-being of humankind.

Table of Contents

Preface i

Foreword iv

Introduction 1

Part One: The Two Traditions 9

1. Modern Ayurveda: Its Sevenfold Nature 11
2. Etiology and Symptomatology of Disease 33
3. Therapeutics 49
4. The Ancient Ayurveda 57
5. The Two Systems Compared 79

Part Two: Symptomatology and Therapeutics in the Ancient Ayurveda 91

6. Symptomatology: Heat, Coldness, Lightness, Heaviness, Dryness, Oiliness, Mixed-Type, and Eighth Disease 93
7. Treating the Diseases 125
8. Western Medicine and the Ancient Ayurveda 153

PART THREE: The Search for Maximum Health and Longevity........................ 161

9. Holistic Health and Its Eight Dimensions....... 163

Conclusion 194

Bibliography.............................. 197

Resources 199

Index.................................. 205

Preface

For the past eighteen years, I have dedicated my life to spreading the study and practice of Ayurveda — the great, universal healing science from India. I have sponsored and supported outstanding Ayurvedic physicians from India, including Dr. Vasant Lad, Dr. Robert Svoboda, and Dr. Sunil Joshi, in addition to publishing and producing twelve books on Ayurveda.

As the producer of this book, I was asked by the author, Ed Tarabilda, to write the Preface. Initially, I hesitated because of the nature of this work. The basic premise of this book is the author's contention that the teachings of Ayurveda which are in existence today are *not* the original Ayurvedic teachings.

The source of modern day Ayurveda is credited to Charaka, who is considered the father of Ayurveda. Ed strongly suggests, and demonstrates through personal case histories over many years and numerous testimonials, that the basis of Ayurveda is not rooted in individual constitution, but rather in seven basic disease tendencies. This is a revolutionary presentation and certainly challenges the approach to Ayurveda which has been followed for the past three thousand years. In fact, all the books I have produced strongly promote the concept of constitution as the basis of Ayurveda.

Therefore, I am going out on a limb to support this work. I do so not because I am rejecting my present understanding and experience with Ayurveda, but in order to give a fresh perspective to allow the reader to reconsider and review his or her understanding and practice of Ayurveda. Personally, I have seen value in using this simple, direct approach to understanding and treating disease. I feel strongly that it deserves attention and investigation by lay people and practitioners of Ayurveda alike. It is important that we not reject any approach, no matter how uncomfortable, because it is contrary to our beliefs and practices. In producing this book, I certainly had to put aside my own experience and even bias as to what I have known to be Ayurveda.

Ultimately, we must all be the authority in our own life, for each of us is fully responsible for ourselves. Therefore, even though what we have heard, read and experienced may be different from what is presented herein, we have a responsibility to determine the truth for ourselves. Personally, I have had reservations about the widely accepted approach of Ayurveda in diagnosing and treating disease, since I have seen that many people do not benefit from the use of Ayurveda for their health issues. Therefore, I am open to considering anything that will support the healing of pain and suffering in humankind.

To accept change, I feel, is humankind's greatest challenge, even though the very nature of life *is* change. It takes courage and a strong willingness to be open to and experience change. I would suggest that you, the reader, approach this book with an open mind and heart, and then determine through your own experience whether it is worthy of consideration as an approach to your personal health and well-being. To me, the only failure in life is not to do.

Lenny Blank
Producer of 13 books on Ayurveda, including
Ayurveda, The Science of Self Healing,
by Dr. Vasant Lad

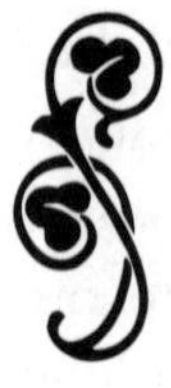

FOREWORD

Ayurveda, the traditional natural healing system of India, is rapidly growing in popularity in the West today. Its system of mind-body medicine considers the physical, psychological and spiritual aspects of healing. Perhaps no other system of medicine has such a practical understanding of all aspects of our being from a cellular level to that of pure consciousness. Ayurveda's series of constitutional types based upon the biological humors provides an individualized approach to healing that is similarly quite profound. Its emphasis on vegetarianism, its connection with Yoga, and its extensive life-style recommendations are other facets of its many sided appeal. Now Ayurveda is regarded as one of the most important systems of alternative medicines available, and one that may hold the key to the future medicine of humanity as we once more recognize the role of consciousness in healing.

After a number of important introductory books on Ayurveda, readers are now being introduced into the deeper aspects of this extraordinary system that covers the whole of life. More complex books are coming out that expand the basic knowledge of Ayurveda in various directions. Through this, the diversity of Ayurveda is being revealed, and we are seeing how different Ayurvedic teachers add their perspectives and bring out different sides of this ocean of knowledge.

Ayurveda Revolutionized is another significant addition to this growing literature of Ayurveda. Yet, the book is also unique in that it does not simply present standard or classical Ayurveda, but asks the reader to challenge and look deeper into the fundamental principles and practices of the entire system. In addition it combines Ayurveda with other Vedic disciplines, like Vedic astrology, that broaden the base of its knowledge.

Readers should note that Ayurveda is not a rigid system following a mechanical order, but a flexible methodology following an organic approach. It is not reducible to any single formulation or to any final presentation. To understand Ayurveda, we must look to its essence and its energies - the powers of body, life, mind and consciousness - and not merely copy or imitate its external forms that must vary along with the abundance of life and the ever fluctuating movement of time. While the diversity of Ayurvedic approaches may appear confusing to beginners in Ayurveda, who may be just learning the ABCs of the system, it is of great relevance to informed students who want to know not only what Ayurveda is but how it works and what lies behind its formulations. *Ayurveda Revolutionized* stimulates such new thinking about Ayurveda and requires such an inquiry in order to appreciate properly.

The author, Edward F. Tarabilda is an original and creative thinker in the Vedic realm, who is not merely content to present standardized information. He looks behind the system and tries to discover what originally gave impetus to it. He seeks to go back to the source. His wide field of knowledge and expertise covers both Ayurveda and its related sister science Vedic Astrology (Jyotish), as well as other aspects of Vedic sciences. For those who are not aware of these connections, Ayurveda shares common terms and approaches with these other Vedic disciplines, particularly astrology, without which the full scope of Ayurvedic practice cannot be understood. An accurate assessment of the birth chart according to the principles of Vedic astrology can add much depth to Ayurvedic treatment.

Tarabilda has done much deep research into these topics over the last twenty years culminating in a whole series of books, of which the present volume is the most recent and most extensive. He adds his own intuitive insight to his study of the Vedic classics and finds much hidden within the teachings that the regular and more superficial glance is bound to miss. In *Ayurveda Revolutionized* he adds another dimension of seeing to Ayurveda and to its related sister science of Vedic astrology. His system of combining Ayurveda with Vedic astrology is both simple and profound. His book is clearly one of the most important new perspectives on Ayurveda to come out in the West. Not only is it significant for Ayurvedic students, it is also relevant for students of Vedic astrology or of Vedic sciences in general.

I have been fortunate enough to know Ed Tarabilda for over twelve years and witness the development in his work. I first met Ed at the Institute of Traditional Medicine in Santa Fe, New Mexico, in early 1983, where he was working with the Ayurvedic program along with Dr. Vasant Lad. In the fall semester of 1983, there was some delay in Dr. Lad returning from India. Ed taught the entire first portion of the program until Dr. Lad returned and continued to teach part of the curriculum throughout the year.

Ed proved to be a good if not exacting teacher, asking his students to think deeply about the subject and not simply accept it at face value. At this point my own background in yogic and Vedic thought was extensive, going back over ten years, including much study of Vedic astrology, but weak on the side of Ayurveda for which I had little access to up to that point. Hence, I was happy to become involved in this Ayurvedic program, one of the first available in the West. Not only did Dr. Lad prove inspirational, helping me to understand this great science, Ed Tarabilda also played a crucial role, for which I will ever be grateful. He made Ayurveda rational and understandable, something to work with on a practical level and not simply stand before silently in awe and accept without knowing why. He also shared my interest in combining Ayurveda with Vedic astrology.

Later in 1984, Ed left Santa Fe to pursue his own personal work. I had little contact with him after that time, but was fortunate enough to meet him on a few occasions and spoken with him several times through the years. Ed began travelling around the country and working with different groups, continuing his research and developing his system.

However, the reader should also note that Tarabilda is rather straightforward in his statements that not everyone is going to share. His claims that the system presented here, what he calls "ancient Ayurveda," may represent the original system of Ayurveda and Vedic astrology, which were originally one, requires further examination. His suggestion that his system is perhaps more accurate than the regular systems of Ayurveda and Jyotish, is yet more controversial, though certainly there is much room for flexibility in the Ayurvedic approach.

But these points aside, whatever the origin of the system Tarabilda presents, it is quite useful and does reflect much insight into both Vedic sciences. It is also very practical and easy to understand in daily application. The book provides a helpful new perspective for all students of Ayurveda or astrology to consider, whether they decide to use it as their primary system, or as a helpful alternative. Let us hope that there will be future books that give us more of the author's wisdom.

David Frawley
Author, *Ayurvedic Healing, Ayurveda And The Mind,*
Co-author, *The Yoga Of Herbs,* Etc.
Santa Fe, NM
March 1997

INTRODUCTION

In recent years a number of Ayurvedic teachers and practitioners, such as Dr. Vasant Lad, Dr. Deepak Chopra, Dr. David Frawley and Dr. Robert Svoboda, have helped make Ayurvedic medicine one of the leading alternative health modalities in the West. Western medicine, with its emphasis on cure rather than prevention, and with its high costs, needs complementary forms of alternative health-care, and Ayurveda fits that need.

Although there are numerous books which set forth the fundamental principles and techniques of modern Ayurvedic medicine, this is the first to present an even more ancient form of Ayurveda, which can be used effectively in conjunction with modern-day Ayurvedic understanding. In fact, I will seek to show that it is this ancient model of Ayurveda which, when combined with the modern model, greatly enhances our ability to prevent and treat disease with precision and effectiveness.

In order to demonstrate this in a useful way, I have used Part One of this book to show the contrast between modern Ayurveda and the ancient Ayurveda. My summary of modern day Ayurveda will be brief, since there are many good books on this subject. If you are already well-grounded in this knowledge, please read at least the last section of the first chapter, entitled "Summing Up."

Part Two of the book seeks to show the symptoms of the seven major diseases according to the ancient Ayurveda, and how to treat each of these seven diseases according to this same ancient model. Part Three teaches us how to prevent each disease-type and how to achieve happy, healthful longevity through the various life strategies gained from the fullness of Vedic knowledge.

I have used the ancient system of Ayurveda, as set forth in this book, in my own practice since the late 1980's. I find it to be a valuable tool for helping people understand how to prevent and cure disease. This ancient approach emphasizes the roots of health and disease, rather than the thousands of disease symptoms which arise from these roots. Such an approach is simple without being simplistic. This system of healing uses the vocabulary of everyday life and experience, so anyone can learn, and even become an expert in this method, without undue effort.

This ancient system of Ayurveda shares much in common with modern Ayurveda, but, as you will see, it uses the basic principles in significantly different ways. This may create some confusion, at first, for those who have been taught the modern day Ayurveda, but in time it will become clear as to how these two approaches are quite complementary and together constitute the complete Ayurveda.

How this Ancient System was Rediscovered

To give a clear picture of how I first cognized, and then objectively confirmed this ancient system of healing, I must engage in a short autobiographical sketch.

My life has had three distinct phases of development: In my youth, spirituality burned brightly within me, but the only avenue open to expressing this spirituality was to become a priest. I entered a Catholic minor seminary for a number of years only to find that Catholicism, as taught in the late Fifties and early Sixties, was inadequate for my needs. I then went through an agnostic stage, and until my mid-thirties was deeply involved in traditional, secular subjects of knowledge. I earned a Bachelor's Degree in Political Science from Loyola University in Chicago and went on to study law, eventually becoming an attorney and a professor of law and government in Springfield, Illinois. It was a conventional and hedonistic life at best!

The second phase began in 1973, when Maharishi Mahesh Yogi, an Indian yogi made popular partly through his association with the Beatles, came through Springfield to address the Illinois legislature on the benefits of Transcendental Meditation (TM). I was a part-time legal advisor to the Illinois Minority Leader, Bill Walsh, at the time, and was quite taken by Maharishi's persona and message. Soon after, I was initiated into TM, and in a short time found my life fundamentally altered by the practice of this technique. All the stress I had accumulated in my brief years of law practice seemed to effortlessly pour out of me through this simple, twice a day, meditative practice.

Before I knew it, I had left my law practice to become a teacher of Transcendental Meditation and eventually found myself deeply involved in what Maharishi called The World Government of the Age of Enlightenment. I became one of the Vice-Presidents of Maharishi International University in Fairfield, Iowa, as well as a professor of law and government. I also took periodic leaves of absence to engage in many long and intensive meditative programs in Europe, one of which culminated in a Master's Degree in the Science of Creative Intelligence, the theoretical aspect of the TM program. Through such programs I found that my consciousness expanded greatly and that I was now sensitive to realms of existence which were inaccessible to me prior to this unfoldment of my awareness.

By the early 1980s, I decided that my research in consciousness should be complemented with a greater knowledge of the physical aspect of life and its relationship to consciousness. But how best to do this? I first did a six month apprenticeship with an herbalist in Austin, Texas. Then I did a six-month herbal studies intensive in California. Finally I completed a two year Ayurvedic studies program with Dr. Vasant Lad in Santa Fe, New Mexico, in one year, and was then asked to stay on and co-teach the first year program with Dr. Lad. After this I opened my own Ayurvedic school in Ojai, California, and later helped found, along with Santosh Krinsky, the Institute for Wholistic Education in Twin Lakes, Wisconsin. This school offers correspondence courses in Ayurveda and other Vedic disciplines. This completed the second significant phase of my life's work.

I could never have predicted what now began to happen in the third phase of my life. Partly, or maybe even completely, as a result of the study and meditation I had engaged in all those years, I began to have very deep, inner cognitions about the nature of life and its unfoldment. Quoting from a brochure which describes my present work in The Art of Multi-Dimensional Living:

> *"The fundamental archetypes of creation spontaneously unfolded in my awareness. These archetypes, or patterns of creative intelligence, displayed themselves as the very fabric of consciousness, each thread unique and precious in itself, yet essential to the whole."*

I also saw that life is a web comprised of eight fields of living. The key to integrating this web into a seamless whole is to understand one's own unique gifts and challenges in each of these eight fields. (These eight fields of living are described at some length in Part Three of this book).

However, as I entered deeply into each field of living and observed what I believe to be its true archetypal form, it became clear to me that many of the Vedic disciplines of knowledge considered today to be original, pure and authentic, are actually so altered from their original form as to be inadequate, and potentially harmful when applied. I found this to be particularly true with regard to Vedic Astrology and Ayurveda, the two most commonly practiced Vedic disciplines. I believe this is true also, to some extent, with regard to Sthapatya Veda (geomancy), Kalpa (ritual), Gandarva Veda (primal music), and the understanding of the Devas (Gods) making up the Vedic cosmology and their relationships to one another. I even discovered major inadequacies in how the Yogas and Darsanas were described, integrated and practiced.

I understood all this through the spiritual cognitions which had unfolded in my awareness. These cognitions, which are even more clear and concise today, relate to the essential nature of each Vedic discipline of knowledge, its relationship to the other disciplines and the intricacies of its practice.

Of course, when a relatively unknown Westerner suggests such a thing, it is bound to be met with considerable skepticism. But I continue to point out the results of my inner investigations in various self-published texts, despite the rancor and confusion it often causes among the Vedic and other ancient mystery traditions.

Since many modern-day people are steeped in scientific materialism in one form or another, they often approach matters of soul and spirit through the physical. Thus, the great interest in Hatha Yoga and Ayurveda. But if this thesis, based on my spiritual cognitions, is correct, modern-day Ayurveda is not the ancient and effective healing system of India, but a later adulteration.

As I point out later in the text, I have found objective confirmation of my cognitions in *Charaka Samhita*, Chapter XXVI, when Charaka makes mention of a system of healing espoused by Varyovida. In my judgment this is the original Ayurvedic system of healing which lost favor when the true science of the stars was no longer practiced and could no longer be used to confirm this original healing system, or show the basis of its practice.

Fortunately, this ancient Ayurveda can be taught without also teaching the ancient true science of the stars I claim to have rediscovered, otherwise all would be lost, because this star science must be discovered in consciousness awareness. It cannot be taught through sheer information like other systems of knowledge. I have written this book to show just how this ancient system of Ayurveda stands on its own and can be used by any practitioner in the same way as any other healing system. I have also included case studies and testimonials to encourage others to begin to use this system of healing in whatever way is useful for them.

Ultimately, it is you the reader experimenting with this model and experiencing its benefits who will determine the reception that this ancient system of healing receives in the field of holistic health. Hopefully, this book serves to shine a new light upon this great and venerable science of life. I offer the following pages in that spirit.

PART ONE

The Two Traditions

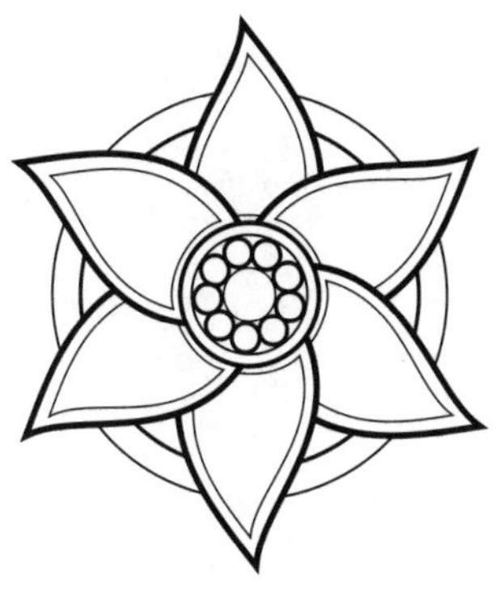

Modern Ayurveda: Its Sevenfold Nature

When we study the laws of nature deeply, we observe that all life has seven levels of existence. In a book entitled *The Reflexive Universe: Evolution of Consciousness*, Arthur M. Young uses scientific investigation to show just how pervasive this sevenfold reality is. He examines in detail how the kingdoms of nature — light, nuclear, atomic, molecular, vegetable, animal and dominion (human) — are sevenfold in nature, and also how each kingdom exhibits seven stages of structure and development: potential, binding, identity, combination, growth, mobility and dominion.

Consequently, it should not surprise us that modern Ayurvedic medicine emphasizes this same sevenfold nature, and views the human physiology as comprised of seven possible body types, seven tissue elements, and seven basic therapeutics, including the science of the seven tastes. But to explain why this is so, we must first explore a threefold paradigm.

According to the Vedas, the knowledge of ancient India, there are three fundamental forces which together weave the manifest universe: the creative force (*rajas*), the preservative force (*sattva*) and the transformative or destructive force (*tamas*). As an example of these principles in action, we can observe how a civilization arises, maintains itself for a while and then falls again, but not without leaving a bedrock for the creation of a new cycle.

At the level of the human physiology, these forces become the three *doshas* (the functional intelligences within the human body) — *Vata, Pitta* and *Kapha*. In terms of the cycle of human existence, Kapha dosha is responsible for the growth of humans to physical maturity (ages 0 - 16); Pitta dosha is responsible for the maintenance of the body in its maturity (16 - 45); and Vata is responsible for the decline of the body (45-death). It is possible that these age groupings can be extended as we achieve greater longevity. For example, it can be argued that the Pitta doshic cycle extends in some people until fifty or fifty-five years of age before the Vata cycle begins.

Constitution

According to the ancient Sankhya philosophy, the human being is made up of many attributes, but the most physical of these attributes are the five elements: ether, air, fire, water and earth. Ether is the most subtle of the elements and the source of the other four. It is pure space, out of which arises the various levels and forms of matter. Air is the equivalent of the gaseous state of matter. Fire is the transformative power of matter which helps change one thing into another. Water is equivalent to the liquid state of matter, and Earth is its solid state.

The three doshas — Vata, Pitta and Kapha — are physical expressions of the five elements. Vata dosha is made up predominantly of ether and air elements. Pitta dosha has a predominance of fire and water elements. Kapha dosha has a predominance of water and earth elements.

Each person will have a preponderance of certain elements in the body when they are born. Some will have more ether and air elements, some more fire and water, and some more water and earth. This preponderance of elements and a particular dosha is called one's constitution.

There are seven possible constitutions:

1. Vata: preponderance of ether and air elements;
2. Pitta: preponderance of fire and water elements;
3. Kapha: preponderance of water and earth elements;
4. Vata-Pitta or Pitta-Vata: less of the earth element;
5. Pitta-Kapha or Kapha-Pitta: less of ether and air elements;
6. Vata-Kapha or Kapha-Vata: less of the fire element; and
7. Vata-Pitta-Kapha: balance among all the elements.

Modern day Ayurveda places great emphasis on the constitution of an individual, and suggests that one should never treat a disease in a way which could aggravate this underlying constitution. Thus, if a practitioner is treating fever in a person who has a Vata-Kapha constitution (cold by nature), the idea is to make sure that the practitioner does not give remedies which cool the body too intensively or for too long because the underlying constitution may become aggravated and cause another disease more severe than the present one.

Modern day Ayurveda further suggests that, most of the time, we are likely to get a disease which corresponds to our constitution. Thus, if we guard against aggravating this constitution, we are less likely to get disease. For example, Vata-types should avoid things that aggravate their doshic balance, like cold, wind, and dryness, as well as all the other things or processes made up predominantly of ether and air elements.

Modern Ayurveda is rooted in a model which sees the principle of excess (like increases like) as primary in disease. Too much ether and air cause a Vata disease, or too much fire and water cause a Pitta disease, etc. In very sick people, excess can fall into deficiency, which will sometimes give symptoms just the opposite of the excess condition. Then one must treat the deficiency until the excess condition reestablishes itself, and then one must again treat that excess condition. Obviously, this shows the complexity that requires professional help during severe illness.

The Attributes

Since these doshas are very subtle substances, we need a special language to talk about them clearly: the language of nature. Charaka and Sushruta, two "ancient" founders and teachers of Ayurveda (the word *ancient* is in quotes because later I will suggest that these are teachers of modern day Ayurveda, not the ancient system), suggest that there are twenty fundamental substances or attributes of any particular substance:

hot and cold	hard and soft
light and heavy	sticky and clear
dry and wet	rough and smooth
acute and dull	gross and subtle
mobile and stable	liquid and solid

Notice that these qualities come in pairs which are opposite one another. So, for example, in order to treat a Vata person who is too cold, give him hot substances, but make sure that these substances are combined with liquids because hot substances can dry out Vata, which is already too dry by nature.

When we apply these twenty qualities to the doshas, we develop an exact, scientific language for speaking about each dosha and its effects. Since these attributes are nothing more than certain combinations of the five elements, and since we have already learned that one dosha has more of certain elements than another, we must conclude that some of these attributes will relate more to one dosha than another.

The attributes relate to the doshas as follows:

VATA: dry, cold, light, unstable, mobile, clear, subtle and rough;

PITTA: hot, light, acute (intense), motile, liquid, oily, and pungent smelling;

KAPHA: heavy, oily, cold, stable, smooth, soft, sticky (viscid), and solid.

Determining Constitution

These attributes can be used to look at the following characteristics in a person: body frame, weight, skin, sweat, hair, eyes, appetite, elimination (stool and urine), stamina, preferred climate, sleep patterns, dreams, sexual habits, fertility, speech, behaviors, emotions, thought processes, memory, and virtually anything else which tends to indicate a preponderance of one or more of the elements and their respective attributes. Since this book is about the ancient model of Ayurveda rather than the modern model, I recommend that readers find a traditional Ayurvedic book for a discussion as to how to evaluate each of the characteristics in terms of their attributes.

Let's take one example to highlight the whole process. If a practitioner is evaluating a client's constitution by looking at her speech patterns, he would expect a Vata person to speak more quickly (mobile), with less passion (cold), in a dry manner (dry), in disjointed or quickly changing ways (unstable), with ease of expression (light), carelessly (rough), but with some subtlety (subtle) and clarity (clear).

A Pitta person would speak in an intense manner (acute), with an irritated or angry inflection (hot) if upset, with passion (pungent smell), in a very precise way (acute), with deep feeling (oily), and with some flair and grace (light and liquid).

A Kapha person would speak slowly (heavy and solid), with dignity (stable), with some passion (oily) and some dispassion (cold), with a steady rhythm (stable and sticky), with softness (soft), and with perseverance (solid and sticky).

From this one example, we can extrapolate as to the other characteristics mentioned above. By following this approach, we learn much more than by just reading and accepting what others say are the bases for determining constitution. Ayurveda is as much an art as it is a science, and it is useful to approach it from both angles.

The Fivefold Division of Each Dosha

When the sages state that the essence of Vata is ether and air, they are suggesting that Vata provides valuable space and cavities in the anatomy (ether), and is also responsible for all types of movement within the physiology.

The movement of Vata can be divided into five types:

1. **PRANA:** This is an inward and downward movement, as when we take air into our lungs or swallow food. This form of Vata resides primarily in the head and brain and is the nerve force (movement) which energizes our whole physiology.
2. **UDANA:** This is an upward and outward movement, as when we exhale, belch or cough. Even speech is under the influence of this energy. This form of Vata is primarily located in the chest and centered in the throat.
3. **SAMANA:** This is a horizontal movement within the body, centered within the stomach and small intestine, where we observe a side-

ways (horizontal) churning as the body seeks to digest food.

4. **VYANA:** This is a circular movement within the body which we can observe when the heart circulates blood throughout the system.
5. **APANA:** This is a downward and outward movement within the body which we can observe through the excretory functions. This form of Vata resides primarily in the colon.

Since Vata is more catabolic or purificatory in nature, and since Apana Vayu is responsible for the removal of waste matter from the system, we can see why this particular form of Vata is of primary importance in the treatment of disease. Constipation is often a major problem for those suffering from an imbalance in the Vata dosha.

When we intentionally or unintentionally interfere with these five natural flows of the vata dosha, then we bring about an imbalance in this dosha. One of the primary ways of doing so is to restrain or suppress natural urges in the body. There are thirteen such urges: 1) to defecate; 2) to pass gas; 3) to urinate; 4) to sneeze; 5) to belch; 6) to yawn; 7) to vomit; 8) to eat; 9) to drink; 10) to cry; 11) to sleep; 12) to pant after exertion; and 13) to ejaculate.

Here we are talking about natural urges — not aberrations due to physical or psychological imbalances and problems. An urge to eat when one is hungry psychologically but not physically can be suppressed without fear of deranging Vata dosha.

The elements of fire and water are the essence of Pitta dosha. Fire is responsible for transformations of all kinds within the body whether mental (digesting information) or physical (digesting food). Metabolism and Pitta go hand-in-hand.

The metabolic transformations of Pitta are of five kinds:

1. **PACHAKA:** Located primarily in the small intestine, this form of Pitta is the fire governing the power of digestion. It is the chief factor in all the inflammatory diseases of Pitta.
2. **SADHAKA:** Located primarily in the brain and heart, this form of Pitta is the fire governing our ability to mentally digest concepts, ideas and beliefs.
3. **BHRAJAKA:** Located primarily in the skin, this form of Pitta is the fire maintaining the health of our skin and its ability to eliminate toxins. It also governs skin tone and texture.
4. **ALOCHAKA:** Located in the eyes, this form of Pitta is the fire governing our visual acuity and the overall health of the eyes.
5. **RANJAKA:** Located primarily in the liver, this form of Pitta is the fire that imparts color and a healthy functioning to the liver, spleen, stomach and small intestine. It gives proper color and consistency to the blood, bile and stool.

Most Pitta problems begin with too much heat in the small intestine. Thus, Pachaka Pitta is primary in treating any disease of Pitta.

The water and earth elements are the essence of Kapha dosha. Kapha dosha is responsible for the growth and stability (earth) of the body as well as its lubrication (water).

There are five forms of Kapha:

1. **TARPAKA:** Located primarily in the brain, spinal cord and heart, this form of Kapha allows the cerebrospinal fluid to form and function normally. Such a condition results in a mental and physical state of peace, harmony and bliss. This form of Kapha also protects memory.
2. **SLESHAKA:** Located primarily in the joints as synovial fluid, this form of Kapha brings lubrication and integrity to the joints and other articulations in the body.
3. **KLEDAKA:** Located primarily in the stomach, this form of Kapha moistens the food as part of the first stage of digestion.
4. **BODHAKA:** Located primarily in the mouth and tongue, this form of Kapha is the moisture which allows us to perceive the sense of taste, which, in turn, signals other parts of the body to prepare for the first stage of the digestive process. This is why those who eat only when they are really hungry tend to have good digestion.
5. **AVALAMBAKA:** Located primarily in the heart and lungs as a protective and lubricating mucous lining, it is also the basic plasma or watery constituent of the body. Since the human body is seventy-five percent water, this constituent gives the body its overall underlying strength and stability.

At times I use the English word "humour" instead of the word *dosha*. This was the ancient Greek word for these same fundamental forces in the physiology, and since we are Westerners, let us sometimes use the term compatible with our own heritage. At the same time, let us not forget the subtlety of the word *dosha*. Dosha means something which can go wrong, or which can fall into error or imbalance. We have already shown the tendency of each dosha to fall into excess and create a particular health problem. So this word has great significance, and we will use it as well.

Other Sites of the Humours

When mentioning the five forms of each humour, I suggested the primary site for each one: Vata in the colon, Pitta in the small intestine and Kapha in the stomach. But each humour also has other sites within the body:

VATA: brain and nervous system, thighs, hips, ears, bones, bladder and organs of touch.

PITTA: stomach, sweat, sebaceous glands, blood, lymph, skin, and the organ of sight.

KAPHA: brain, joints, chest, throat, head, pancreas, sides, lymph, fat, nose, tongue, and the organ of taste.

Aggravation of the Humours

When these humours become excessive, they create certain symptoms:

VATA: emaciation, debility, constipation, coldness, dizziness, tremors, sleep impairment, confusion, depression and incoherence.

PITTA: fever, inflammation, hunger, thirst, insomnia, burning sensations, anger, and a yellowish tint to the skin, eyes, stool and urine.

KAPHA: nausea, depression, heaviness, lethargy, chills, excess sleep, cough with mucus and phlegm, difficult breathing, white coloring, edema, and poor or slow digestion.

If the excess condition becomes severe enough, the person can fall into deficiency and then his symptoms will often appear to be the opposite of his basic humoural imbalance. For example, when Vata becomes deficient, the person may develop a fever and have loose stool. There may also be lethargy and heaviness. This could easily be misdiagnosed as a Pitta or Kapha problem, or a combination of both. Fortunately, these conditions are not common, and generally occur only in seriously ill people. So, with seriously ill people, it is important to be very careful with diagnosis.

The Seven Dhatus or Tissue Elements

Just as there are seven possible basic constitutions, there are also seven basic tissue elements within the physiology. Each tissue, until the seventh, has another tissue related to it which lies deeper in the physiology. This deeper tissue takes nutrients from the more surface ones. Thus, the more we use the energy and nutrients of the deeper tissues, the more we potentially stress the more surface tissues, because they must replenish the deeper tissues with their own energy and nutrients. On the other hand, a failure to provide the deeper tissues with basic nourishment from the surface level tissue is also a cause of disease.

This first tissue level is called *rasa dhatu* — plasma, lymph or sap. It consists of the primal nutrients from digested food which is then circulated into the blood. The blood is the second tissue layer as we move deeper into the physiology. Healthy blood helps form muscle tissue, the third dhatu, which, in turn, helps form the fourth tissue, called adipose tissue. Adipose tissue helps form bone tissue (the fifth level). Bone tissue helps form bone marrow and nerve tissue (sixth level). Finally, bone marrow helps form the seventh, deepest and last tissue — reproductive tissue.

Thus, poor nutrition of the rasa dhatu level damages the deeper tissue levels. And, as controversial as this may be, Ayurveda suggests that excess depletion of the reproductive fluid, especially in males, can also tax the system as well. Reproductive fluid is the essence of all the other tissues, and its excessive loss places great demand on the other tissues to replace that loss. Even excess demands on the nerve tissue can create similar crises in the other tissues since it is the second deepest tissue. Consequently, ill-health can arise from either the shallow or deep end of the tissue layers.

Tissue Functions

Another way of understanding the tissues is by their function in the body:

Rasa dhatu nourishes the physiology and helps maintain menstruation and lactation in the female. This is why proper nourishment is so important for both the conception of children and while nursing. This dhatu helps maintain a love of self.

Rakta Dhatu provides oxygenation and, thus, life and vitality to the system, particularly the blood vessels and muscle tendons. It helps us feel vital and enthusiastic.

Mamsa Dhatu covers the vital organs as well as providing movement and strength to the joints. It gives us our sense of physical security, and helps maintain the flat muscles and skin.

Meda Dhatu lubricates and oils the tissues and helps maintain subcutaneous fat and proper sweating. It creates a feeling of psychological warmth and caring.

Asthi Dhatu gives support to the whole body and helps us maintain our sense of balance. It also helps us maintain proper teeth, hair and nail growth.

Majja Dhatu gives us a sense of substance and confidence by filling the spaces in the bones. It also relates to the nervous system and the proper functioning of motor and sensory impulses. It helps maintain lachrymal secretions.

Shukra Dhatu maintains the reproductive organs and functions, and gives us our sense of creativity.

Malas or Waste Products

The concept of malas is another important one in Ayurveda. There are three basic waste products produced from body structure and processes: feces, urine, and sweat. The proper elimination of these waste products is vital to health.

It is not proper to think of these substances as just waste. Each of these by-products has important, positive physiological functions in the body. For example, the colon absorbs many useful nutrients from the feces once they are formed. In other words, nutrition is not restricted to the digestive processes which take place in the small intestine and stomach. Proper sweating through the skin helps relieve the kidneys of some of its burden of purification, and proper urine flow keeps the skin from having to eliminate toxins beyond its capacity as well.

The condition of each of the three malas, particularly feces and urine, are important when we seek to distinguish whether a dosha is deranged with *Ama* or without Ama. Ama is a technical term which means toxin. When digestion is inadequate at any stage or level, toxins form in the system. When a dosha is deranged and Ama is also present, it is called *Sama* Vata, Pitta or Kapha. When a dosha is deranged without the presence of Ama, it is called *Nirama* Vata, Pitta or Kapha. There is a very good discussion of Sama and Nirama conditions and their symptoms in *The Yoga of Herbs* by Dr. David Frawley and Dr. Vasant Lad. Ama tends to form when a person's *Agni* is deranged.

Agni

Agni is the biological fire which transforms foreign substances into homogenous substances. When you eat spinach and transform it into muscle and flesh, then you are using the force of Agni. We can even think of the process of digestion and metabolism as a sevenfold process: 1) Ingesting; 2) Digesting; 3) Absorbing; 4) Transporting; 5) Transforming; 6) Utilizing; and 7) Excreting. Such a perspective tends to come from either modern medicine or from a deep appreciation of the ancient science of the stars rather than from modern day Ayurveda.

According to Charaka, strength, beauty, and longevity are all due primarily to the normal functioning of Agni. A complete discussion of Agni would require a book in itself, since the processes of digestion and metabolism take place first in the small intestine (*Jathara* Agni), then in the intermediate metabolism (*Bhutagni*) through some of the major digestive organs, and finally through cellular metabolism (*Dhatvagni*). What is amazing is that a science many thousands of years old could have such a complete understanding of modern chemistry and physiology, although certainly expressed in different terms.

Each dosha tends to have a type of Agni functioning. Vata tends to variable Agni, with the digestion being sometimes good and sometimes bad. Pitta tends to high Agni with excessive appetite and the development of inflammatory problems in the digestive system. Kapha tends to slow Agni, which often results in food turning to fat all too easily. When these tendencies do not take place, then one has balanced Agni with good digestion.

There is also a condition known as low Agni, in which a person has trouble digesting food because the gastric fire is not strong enough to handle normal quantities of food. Ama is easily formed from such a condition and, thus, it is a serious problem.

The Four Essential Principles

A study of modern day Ayurveda is a study of Doshas, Dhatus, Malas and Agnis. These four principles describe the basic structures and processes within Ayurvedic theory and practice. Sometimes there is confusion as to where structure or substance ends and process begins. For example, is Agni a subtle substance like the grosser substances of tissues and waste matter, or is it merely an aspect of Pitta dosha? Is Kapha dosha more of a substance than Pitta or Vata dosha? Is Pitta dosha more a substance like Kapha or more a process like Vata? There are always self-proclaimed authorities eager to give definite answers to such questions, but we should realize that life is one whole and, at a certain level, processes and substances interact and merge in ways beyond rational scrutiny. Thus, to stay open to this more subtle view supports understanding.

Bodily Systems (*Srotas*)

Another way of summing up the previous material is to list all the possible channels in the body through which the various substances and processes (doshas, dhatus, malas and agnis) either flow or are carried out. There are sixteen Srotas or channels in modern day Ayurveda.

Three channels relate primarily to the three doshas:

1. *Pranavaha Srotas* — the channel that relates to breath and the carrying of Prana. It is composed primarily of the respiratory system, although it must include the heart as well. This channel is related archetypally to Vata dosha.
2. *Annavaha Srotas* — the food channel and digestive system. This channel is related archetypally to Pitta dosha.
3. *Ambhuvaha Srotas* — the channel that carries water and regulates water metabolism. It is related archetypally to Kapha dosha.

Seven channels relate to the seven tissues in the body:

4. *Rasavaha Srotas* — the lymph channels originating in the heart and its vessels.
5. *Raktavaha Srotas* — the blood channels originating in the liver and spleen.
6. *Mamsavaha Srotas* — the muscle channels originating in the muscle and skin.
7. *Medavaha Srotas* — the adipose channels originating in the kidneys and momentum.
8. *Asthivaha Srotas* — the bone channels originating in the fat and the hips.
9. *Majjavaha Srotas* — the marrow and nerve channels originating in the bones and joints.
10. *Shukravaha Srotas* — the reproductive channels originating in the testes or uterus.

Two special channels exist in the female, which are related to, but separate from, the reproductive channels:

11. *Artavaha Srotas* — menstrual channels.
12. *Stanyavaha Srotas* — channels that carry breast milk.

Three additional channels relate to the Malas:

13. *Svedavaha Srotas* — sweat carrying channels originating in the adipose tissue and hair follicles.
14. *Purishavaha Srotas* — feces carrying channels originating in the colon and rectum.
15. *Mutravaha Srotas* — urine carrying channels originating in the kidneys and bladder.

Finally there is a last srota:

16. *Manovaha Srotas* — the channels that carry thought in the mind. Obviously these channels exist throughout the entire body.

Thus, you can see how doshas, dhatus and malas exist as channels within the body. Since there is no Srota directly related to Agni, we can conclude that it is more of a doshic process than a substance. Nevertheless, Agni is one of the four main pillars upon which Ayurveda is constructed and practiced.

Nyaya Darsana, the first system of Indian philosophy, suggests that there are sixteen ways to approach any object of knowledge; if one uses all sixteen approaches, then one is assured of complete truth. This principle is reflected in the sixteen Srotas.

We should also be aware of the fact that the Chinese system of healing uses fourteen major channels for promoting health and healing disease. It has been assumed in recent centuries that the Chinese system is totally separate from the Ayurvedic one. In the past few years, several books have come out seeking to show the interactions between the two systems. One such book, *The Lost Secrets Of Ayurvedic Acupuncture* by Dr. Frank Ros, highlights common aspects of both systems.

Subtle Anatomy and Physiology

Because anatomy and physiology have a relationship to psychology and spirituality, some Vedic sages have set forth the subtle corollaries to Vata, Pitta and Kapha doshas. Subtle Vata is *Prana*, the life force within the human. Subtle Pitta is *Tejas*, the very subtle fire which governs all transformations and transmutations within the human personality. And subtle Kapha is *Ojas*, the essence of bodily substance and integrity. Together these three forces unite body, mind and spirit. Such language is helpful for understanding the Vedic descriptions of the vital body — the subtle energy body related to the physical body — and how this body is described as having three major conduits called *Nadis* and seven major plexuses called *Chakras*.

A good description and discussion of this more subtle aspect of Ayurveda is given by Robert Svoboda in his book *Prakruti: Your Ayurvedic Constitution*, and in a book which he co-authored, *Tao and Dharma*. Dr. Vasant Lad, in his now classic primer *Ayurveda: The Science of Self-Healing*, also discusses these topics in his chapter on longevity.

Discussions on these more subtle aspects of Ayurveda help tie material considerations to psychological and spiritual ones. Nevertheless, these subtle principles can hardly be considered primary ones in the daily practice of Ayurveda.

Summing Up

The four principles that must be thoroughly understood in order to be applied to all aspects of anatomy and physiology, health and disease are: the three Doshas; the seven Dhatus; the three Malas; and the various forms and levels of Agni.

The language that is used to discuss these four principles is the language of the twenty attributes: heavy/light, slow/sharp, cold/hot, oily/dry, slimy/rough, dense/liquid, soft/hard, static/mobile, subtle/gross and cloudy/clear. Note that these are slightly different words from the ones I first used to describe these attributes. This is to help develop some flexibility in how these qualities are viewed.

Actual diagnosis and treatment takes place through one or more of the sixteen channels of the body previously discussed.

The three doshas become important in the context of physiological constitution and the seven doshic configurations which make up the science of constitutional typing.

An idea that is essential to modern day Ayurveda is knowing one's constitutional type, and managing it, according to the rules of Ayurveda, as the best way to prevent disease and achieve longevity. This is why a modern day Ayurvedic physician like Robert Svoboda can make the statement in *Tao and Dharma: Chinese Medicine and Ayurveda*,: "Since Ayurveda, in general, focuses more on understanding and treating constitutional types, whereas Chinese medicine predominantly addresses specific disease patterns, these two approaches towards healthy living are potentially complementary."

A second essential idea is that one is most prone to the diseases which are related to one's body type. A predominantly Kapha body type is most likely to get Kapha diseases, even though there is the possibility of such a person getting a Pitta or Vata disease. If the Kapha person does get a Pitta or Vata disease, then one must be careful to treat that disease in a way that does not aggravate the underlying constitutional type (Kapha in this case). Thus, Dr. David Frawley and Dr. Vasant Lad, in *Yoga of Herbs,* state: "But for deeper and more chronic diseases, for long term treatment, knowledge of the constitution is essential for a complete and effective therapy."

The ancient model of Ayurveda does not accept or use the first essential idea of modern day Ayurveda, nor does it completely accept all aspects of the second idea or strategy. Why this is so will become clear when we discuss the ancient model. The ancient Ayurveda accepts all the sevenfold paradigms of modern Ayurveda, but adds a new and possibly deeper sevenfold paradigm of its own.

What causes a particular humour to go out of balance? If we can know that, then we can prevent that imbalance from arising in the first place. This brings us to the etiology of disease.

The Etiology of Disease

When most people think of the causes of disease, they think in terms of common-sense principles: stay out of the cold and wet weather if you don't want to catch a cold, or don't overeat if you don't want a belly-ache. Although such ideas are useful, they hardly satisfy the philosopher, scientist or physician. Properly understood, the causes of disease are sevenfold:

1. Genetic – due to defects in the mother's or father's genes;
2. Congenital – due to errors in conduct of the pregnant mother;
3. Constitutional – due to aggravation of the doshas in the constitution one is born with;
4. Traumatic – due to external and internal injuries;
5. Seasonal disorders – due to the failure to adapt to seasonal changes;
6. Infectious and spiritual – due to epidemic or pandemic influences, or acts of God; and
7. Natural diseases – due to normal or premature aging.

To understand how any of these causes arise, we must engage in a further study of the nine fundamental, material causes of all composite things. This is one of the major subjects analyzed through *Vaisheshika Darsana*, the second system of Indian Philosophy. According to this system of knowledge there are nine fundamental substances and causal essences in the universe: 1) earth, 2) water, 3) fire, 4) air, 5) ether, 6) direction, 7) time, 8) mind and 9) soul. The first five elements relate to the organs of cognition which smell, taste, see, touch and hear. These organs can be underused or overused and misused, which aggravates one or more of the humours in the body.

The Five Organs of Cognition

1. Smell: It is overuse to smell sharp, pungent, overly perfumed odors; it is underuse not to smell anything at all; it is misuse to smell odors which are putrid, toxic, poisonous or decayed.
2. Taste: It is overuse to indulge in overeating; it is underuse to fast too long or too often; it is misuse not to follow the various Ayurvedic rules of dietetics. These rules are available in many modern Ayurvedic texts.
3. Sight: It is overuse to stare excessively at overly bright objects; it is underuse not to exercise the eyes at all or to remain in darkness for too long a period of time; it is misuse to stare at overly small or distant objects for too long, or to stare at horrible sights.

4. Touch: It is overuse to expose oneself to too much cold and heat, or to engage in massage too often; it is underuse to never expose oneself to massage or other tactile stimuli; it is misuse to let the body touch uneven surfaces for too long, or to touch unclean things.
5. Hearing: It is overuse to listen to overly loud or stimulating sounds; it is underuse to avoid sound; it is misuse to listen to sounds which are harsh, terrifying or afflicting in some way.

The Organs of Action

The five elements also relate to the five organs of action: elimination, generation (sexual procreation), locomotion, grasping, and speaking. The suppression or forced excitation of any of these organs of action can seriously derange one or more of the doshas. For example, if someone doesn't speak for a certain number of years, he may lose the ability to speak altogether. If one doesn't exercise, one loses muscle strength and conditioning. If one speaks or exercises too much, or misuses these organs of action, this also causes ill health. If one suppresses any of the thirteen natural urges discussed earlier, then one deranges Vata dosha.

One can not only misuse the body, one can also misuse speech. Language which is insinuating, untrue, quarrelsome, unpleasant, untimely, incoherent, unhelpful, or which creates a bad feeling in the environment is also a cause of disease.

Some of these causes may not be potent causes, so they are often dismissed as insignificant. But that is not always the case, and that is why they are mentioned in the ancient texts.

Direction

There are eight directions: north, south, east, west, northwest, southwest, southeast and northeast. There are also eight directions to our life, called fields of living. When our approach to any of these eight fields is frustrated, it can affect our health and longevity. These fields are: 1) Spiritual life; 2) Wealth; 3) Dharma or caste nature; 4) Creative play; 5) Interpersonal relationships; 6) Professional life; 7) Mental health; and 8) Physical health. This topic will be examined in detail in Part Three of this book.

Time

There are four important time factors in discussing the etiology of disease and the vitiation of the doshas:

1. Time of season — Vata dosha is aggravated in the dry, windy and cold late autumn. Pitta dosha is aggravated in the hot summer and early fall. Kapha dosha is aggravated in the cold, damp winter and early spring. For different countries with their different climates and seasons, these rules will vary somewhat. If one fails to alter the diet and regimen according to the season, one is likely to aggravate the humour related to that season.
2. Time of day or night — Vata dosha becomes easily aggravated from 3 - 7 a.m. and p.m.,

Kapha dosha from 7 - 11 a.m. and p.m., and Pitta dosha from 11 - 3 a.m. and p.m.

3. Time of digestion — Kapha predominates during the first predigestive phase after eating; Pitta predominates during the digestive phase and Vata predominates during the assimilative phase. How long each phase lasts varies from person to person, but the first phase is usually an hour or so, the second phase four to six hours, and the third phase eight to twelve hours.
4. Time of life — Kapha dosha is dominant from birth to sixteen; Pitta from sixteen to forty-five; and Vata from forty-five until death. Since the first phase is quite anabolic, the middle balanced, and the last quite catabolic, one must follow certain rules during each period. Many of these rules relate to conserving one's strength after entering the third phase.

Mind

Individuals not only have physical constitutions, they also have mental constitutions. There are three basic types of mental disposition: 1)*sattvic*; 2)*rajasic*; and 3)*tamasic*.

The sattvic mental constitution has the qualities of purity and fineness. It does not, by itself, promote disease, but sattva never appears in pure form — it is always tainted by rajas and tamas, which do produce disease. Thus, until someone is fully spiritually enlightened, he will never have a totally sattvic mind. There are seven sattvic sub-types, according to *Sushruta Samhita*. How to apply the various sub-types in practical ways is not taught in modern Ayurveda. The rajasic mental constitution has the qualities of action and desire. It has six sub-types, according to *Sushruta Samhita*. The tamasic mental constitution has the qualities of inertia, solidity and resistance. It has three sub-types, according to *Sushruta Samhita*.

Those of a predominantly rajasic or tamasic mental constitution will tend to indulge in one or more of the seven negative emotions: pride, cruelty (withholding love), anger, self-centeredness, attachment to purity, procrastination, and fear and insecurity. These negative emotions can vitiate any of the doshas, although Vata is more related to fear, insecurity and self-centeredness, Pitta to anger and pride, and Kapha to the withholding of love, procrastination and attachment. Others have defined the seven sins as: gluttony, greed, envy, lust, pride, wrath and slothfulness. In any case, all these negative emotions can trigger the advent of disease.

Soul

Pragya Paradha is defined as the fundamental ignorance of who we really are, or what we are not. This is considered to be the primary cause of all disease because ignorance of our true nature leads to mental and behavioral aberrations and other mistakes of the intellect, which directly or indirectly cause disease. It is for this reason that Yoga is considered a necessary corollary of Ayurveda.

Additional Insights

Thus, we see how the nine causes of Vaisheshika's philosophy relate to Ayurveda. Another way of talking about etiology is to emphasize that disease can be exogenous (externally caused) or endogenous (internally caused). It can also be somatic (related to the physical constitution) or psychic (related to the mental constitution).

Probably the easiest way to approach the subject of etiology of disease is to remember the attributes which relate to each humour, and to realize that too much of that attribute in any form is the cause of disease. For example, Vata is too dry by nature, so dry wind, dry sun, dry foods, or medicines which dry the body can all aggravate Vata. Even emotions like fear and anxiety can dry out the body and be a precipitating factor for disease. For further discussion of this subject, please consult Ayurvedic texts.

One final point: the ancient Ayurveda accepts all that modern Ayurveda teaches regarding the general etiology of disease, except that it does not agree with the idea that aggravation of the innate constitution is a primary cause of disease.

J. B. (Los Angeles, CA):

"I was told that I was suffering from a classic Pitta aggravation due to my predominantly Pitta constitution getting out of balance. I often suffered from tense, sore muscles with heat radiating from them, or so it seemed. But the program to reduce Pitta and the fire element in my system didn't seem to work. I found no relief from my symptoms. I was then exposed to the more ancient model of Ayurveda, with the idea that dryness was the fundamental disease paradigm needing treatment through oleation therapy. I was a little skeptical at first, especially since modern Ayurveda suggests that oleation therapy would exacerbate my condition, but it worked. I am now symptom free and I also have a lot more energy."

CASE STUDY

S. C. came to me for a health consultation. His disease tendency — using the ancient Ayurvedic model — was the disease of lightness. This caused him to become easily confused and "spaced-out," even as regards his own ailments. He was also a victim of periodic allergies and hyper-sensitivities. One practitioner of the modern Ayurveda said that such symptoms were a classic example of Vata derangement and treated him accordingly, without relief. Another Ayurvedic doctor suggested that Pitta was the culprit and gave him bitter herbs to reduce the heat in his system. This seemed to aggravate his condition even more.

That bitters would cause an aggravation of his condition is easily explained according to the ancient Ayurveda. Such a person needs primarily sweet tasting foods and herbs and all other forms of nourishing therapy. He was put on this program and has shown steady progress, except when he works and/or plays too hard and aggravates the attribute of lightness. Then he must apply himself to nourishing and resting his body and mind until he has brought his exaggerated catabolic tendency under control.

Symptomatology of Disease

When we search for an excess in any of the twenty basic attributes in any of the sixteen channels of the body, then we are in the realm of symptomatology of disease. This search is called the *science of diagnostics*. For example, if you are examining pranavaha srota, and respiration is very rapid, slow, shallow or deep, agitated or interrupted, or associated with abnormal sounds, pain or feelings, then we can assume pathological change in that srota due to the vitiation of one of the doshas.

Determining which humour is at fault is called *differential diagnosis*. In David Frawley's excellent book, *Ayurvedic Healing*, there is a section under each disease called "Differentiation." Certain symptoms indicate a particular humour is excessively high. For example, if one has a dry, hacking cough without expectoration, it indicates a Vata lung derangement. If there is a lot of mucus and phlegm, then Kapha is involved. If the mucus is infectious, then Pitta is involved. It is even possible that all three humours are deranged at once.

The difficulty with this modern Ayurvedic approach is that it is quite complex. On the other hand, the ancient Ayurveda suggests that there are only seven major diseases, and that all other diseases mentioned in modern Ayurveda or modern Western medicine are nothing more than symptoms of one of these seven underlying diseases. Without this necessary simplification in understanding, people are often left in confusion about what is causing what.

I frequently encounter people who are using modern day Ayurveda or Chinese medicine — either on their own or through alternative practitioners — who really don't know what their disease tendency actually is. They will say: "My lungs and kidneys are off," or "I've been muscle tested and it has shown I have weak spleen and stomach energy," or "I think Vata is deranged," when it is only too apparent from the ancient system of Ayurveda that they are not clear. I would submit that proper diagnosis has eluded them because the Eastern and Western models of disease have complicated the issue. That, at least, is the thesis of this book.

How does modern Ayurveda look at diagnostics? As we might expect, the approach is very comprehensive. Based upon the knowledge acquired from Ayurvedic authorities, we must use all the sense organs (except for the sense of taste, according to Charaka) as methods of diagnosis:

1. Examination by Tactile Sense (Palpation):
   - Through examination of the pulses.
   - Through palpation of various parts of the body:
     - hot and cold
     - moist and dry
     - rough or smooth
     - tense or relaxed
     - soft or hard
   - Other techniques used by physicians and body workers to determine health and disease.
2. Examination with the Eye (Observation):
   - Through observing the forms, proportions, shapes, colors and luster of body from the

top of the head all the way down to the tips of the toes.

Constitutional examination (*prakruti*).

Determination of present humoural balance (*vikruti*).

3. Examination with the Ear (Auscultation):

   Voice — sounds, intestinal sounds, the sounds of joints when the patient moves, cardiac or respiratory sounds, etc.

4. Examination through Smell: the whole body, but especially the three malas when possible.

5. Examination through Taste:

   Prohibited — probably because of sanitary reasons. Nevertheless, there were some ancient physicians who could diagnose through tasting any of the three malas — repugnant as that may be to modern-day people.

One should use the above-mentioned senses to examine all sixteen channels in the body as well as the overall body build and measurements. One should pay particular attention to pulse, eye, lip, tongue and nail diagnosis, and query the patient about the functioning of the three malas. In fact, we not only want to examine each of the sixteen srotas, we also want to question the patient about them.

Examination and questioning are the two major diagnostic methods. In asking the patient questions, one should focus on: 1) chief complaints and how long they have existed; 2) possible causes of the present illness; 3) past illnesses; 4) family history; and 5) personal history relevant to the present complaints. *Ayurveda: The Science of Self-Healing*, by Dr. Vasant Lad, gives many practical diagnostic techniques in some detail.

In doing diagnostics or studying any other Ayurvedic text on symptomatology, keep in mind that, in order to keep this subject from becoming overly complex, the Ayurvedic sage, Charaka, suggested an eight-fold examination: 1) the pulse; 2) the urine; 3) the feces; 4) the tongue; 5) the skin; 6) the voice; 7) the eyes; and 8) the face. Using the various diagnostic techniques to evaluate these eight aspects of the anatomy and physiology will yield excellent results. It is this eight-fold examination which I will emphasize when discussing the symptomatology of disease according to the ancient Ayurveda.

No matter how much information the practitioner gathers, he or she will still have to draw inferences from what the person says, or from what the practitioners can observe about themselves in the case of self-diagnosis and treatment. For example, in trying to determine how strong a digestion a person has, the practitioner must ask him many questions about when, where, and how he eats, and what the after-effects are. Even after all these questions, inferences must still be made.

This is why the whole science of diagnosis is a combination of three factors: the study of the basic medical texts; direct perception and questioning of the patient; and drawing inferences about the patient's condition and the causes of his condition.

Pathogenesis

One must be able not only to diagnose the nature of the disease, but also to know the stage of the disease. Ayurveda discusses six stages of disease:

1. Accumulation — Vata begins to increase in the colon, Pitta in the small intestine, and Kapha in the stomach. The causes can be any of those discussed in the chapter on the etiology of disease.
2. Aggravation — Vata, Pitta or Kapha increase in each of their respective sites even more. The symptoms of each deranged dosha magnify.
3. Overflow — The humours now overflow and spread throughout the body. They tend to localize once again in weak spots in the physiology, bringing about the fourth state.
4. Displacement — The humour(s) lodge in weak spots where they begin to cause specific disease symptoms.
5. Manifestation — Symptoms are so clear that the disease paradigm can now be identified with certainty.
6. Flowering — Most or all the major attributes of the humour related to the disease will be in evidence. Complications of the disease may also take place, and these complications can often be worse than the original disease, i.e. gangrene in diabetes.

People who are very sensitive to their bodies, either through meditation or some other psycho-physiological training, can become aware of these stages of disease as they happen. Such people are likely to take preventive action while a disease is in the accumulation stage, thus preventing the second stage of increase or further stages from developing.

The Three Pathways of Disease

We can understand the stages of disease from yet another Ayurvedic paradigm — the three pathways:

1. The Inner Pathway: the gastro-intestinal tract (stomach, small intestine and large intestine.) Even though called "inner," this is the most superficial of all the pathways, and any disease is easiest to treat when in this first pathway.
2. The Outer Pathway: consisting of the first two tissue systems — lymph and blood and the circulatory system as a whole. This is the second deepest pathway, and disease tendencies in this pathway are still easier to treat than those which have reached the deepest pathway. Skin rashes, lymphatic problems or circulatory disorders are examples of disease symptoms in this pathway.
3. The Central Pathway: consisting of the last five dhatus — muscle, fat, bone, marrow and reproductive tissue. Often it is a Vata disease that affects this third pathway, and such Vata diseases are very difficult to treat.

Cancer is a sixth-stage disease that involves all three pathways and all three humours. Thus, it is very difficult to treat.

If we were more sensitive to these three pathways, we could often avoid disease. Take the case of the typical cold or flu. It usually starts with the digestion becoming weak (first pathway). If a person immediately heeds that warning and takes in no food for twenty-four hours, he often doesn't get the cold or flu, or he gets a very mild case of it. If he goes ahead and eats anyway, the illness comes on in full force. Nature is like a kind mother, but we don't always want to listen to her advice!

All diseases are due to either under-nourishment (catabolic process) or over-nourishment (anabolic process). Under-nourishment starves all the tissues in the body and over-nourishment weakens the agni (like putting too much fuel on a fire) and clogs the system with toxins (ama). This particular understanding of the twofold nature of disease is extremely important in the ancient Ayurveda, as will be explained in the following chapters.

Basically, diagnostics and symptomatology are the same in the ancient Ayurveda as in modern Ayurveda, except that the ancient model emphasizes root diseases rather than their many leaves and branches.

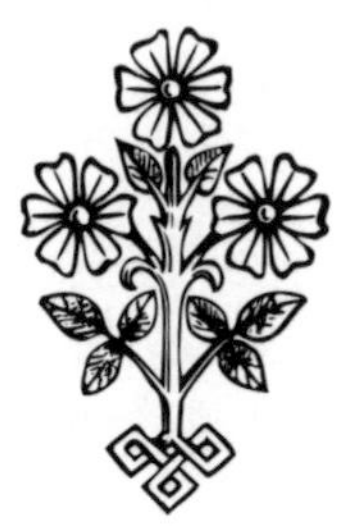

Therapeutics

There are eight major clinical disciplines in Ayurveda: 1) Geriatrics; 2) Virilization or Fertilization Therapy; 3) Internal Medicine; 4) Surgery; 5) Eye, Ear, Nose and Throat Diseases; 6) Toxicology; 7) Psychiatry; and 8) Gynecology, Obstetrics and Pediatrics. In all of these disciplines, one tries first to prevent disease. If that fails, then one seeks to cure the disease through the respective techniques developed in each of the eight disciplines.

Preventive Measures

Preventive measures are discussed in more detail in Part Three of this book, but in general they consist of:

1. Appropriate **daily routines**, such as washing the mouth and brushing the teeth regularly; putting oil drops in the ears, nose, and on the head; scraping the tongue; exercising regularly; and other forms of personal hygiene. Government regulation of hygiene i.e. water, sewage etc., also plays a major role in modern disease prevention.

2. The use of **rejuvenating and virilizing agents** to enhance longevity, increase immunity to disease, improve mental functioning and add vitality and luster to the body.
3. The development of effective **life strategies** for holistic living in each of the eight fields of life. Of the eight fields, the field of spiritual life is the most important because it combats the fundamental ignorance which is the root cause of all disease.

Curative Measures

Curative measures are fourfold:

1. INTERNAL MEDICINE: Which in turn has two major types of procedures — Internal Purification and Curative Treatment:

    (a) **Internal Purification**: This is also known as *Panchakarma*, translated as "the five purifications." The first purification is emesis (vomiting), the second is purgation, the third is medicated enema, the fourth is nasal administration of herbs, and the last is blood-letting. In *Ayurveda: Secrets of Healing*, Maya Tiwari gives a complete guide to Panchakarma treatment, as does another excellent book, *Ayurveda and Panchakarma* by Dr. Sunil V. Joshi.

    In my view, modern Ayurveda uses Panchakarma in ways which can be counterproductive for some people. One of the benefits of the ancient Ayurvedic model is that it uses Panchakarma in more precise ways than modern Ayurveda.

(b) **Curative Treatment**: Through dietetics, medicinal substances such as herbs and metals, and various forms of treatment through any of the other four senses — sound therapy, color therapy, aromatherapy, massage and marma point therapy. Some of these therapies could be thought of as part of the next category of medicine, external medicine.

Ayurveda & Aromatherapy by Drs. Light and Bryan Miller is an excellent book on Ayurvedic Aromatherapy. *Ayurveda: Secrets of Healing*, by Maya Tiwari, not only explores Panchakarma, but also Ayurvedic massage and marma-point therapy. Deepak Chopra and Maharishi Ayurvedic practitioners use a technique they call "Primal Sound Therapy" to cure disease and promote health. Many of the Ayurvedic therapies have been explored quite extensively here in the West.

2. EXTERNAL MEDICINE: Therapies are applied to the external part of the body, whether pastes, oils, baths, massages or other forms of physio-therapeutic treatment. *Ayurvedic Beauty Care* by Melanie Sachs is an excellent book for learning how to invoke or enhance natural beauty through the principles and techniques of Ayurveda.
3. SURGERY: This was once a highly-developed division within Ayurveda, but it is no longer so. Western technology has usurped the field.
4. PSYCHOSOMATIC MEDICINE. This form of medicine will be explored in Part Three of the

book as part of preventive and rejuvenative therapy.

One of the most important parts of curative treatment is dietetics, herbology and homeopathics. Modern Ayurveda recognizes homeopathy in principle, but seldom uses it in practice. The ancient Ayurveda used it extensively, especially the seven metals.

For those who are unfamiliar with the distinction between allopathic and homeopathic medicine: Allopathic medicine treats like with unlike, such as a disease of heat with cold substances or a disease of coldness with hot substances; Homeopathic medicine treats like with like, such as the disease of heat with hot substances. Although these homeopathic substances are etheric in nature, they signal the body to reduce heat naturally through a message which the immune system can recognize. In the example at hand, the message would be, "I'm too hot!"

The Science of Taste

Modern Ayurveda uses the science of taste to help balance the humours, whether the balancing is through food or medicinal substances like herbs, metals or homeopathics. There are six major tastes in Ayurveda: sweet, sour, salty, bitter, pungent and astringent. Some tastes aggravate or calm Vata, some aggravate or calm Pitta and some Kapha. This is because each taste is made up primarily of certain elements:

1. sweet = water and earth
2. sour = earth and fire

3. salty = water and fire
4. bitter = ether and air
5. pungent = fire and air
6. astringent = earth and air

Since Vata is primarily ether and air, and Pitta is primarily fire and water, and Kapha is water and earth, it stands to reason that certain tastes aggravate each humour and calm each humour as follows:

Vata — bitter, pungent and astringent aggravate; sweet, sour and salty calm; Pitta — pungent, sour and salty taste aggravate; sweet, bitter and astringent calm; and Kapha — sweet, sour and salty aggravate; bitter, pungent and astringent calm.

Most basic books on Ayurveda go into the subject of dietetics in some detail, but I think *The Ayurvedic Cookbook*, by Amadea Morningstar with Urmila Desai, is one of the best because of the great detail with which she discusses this subject. *The Yoga of Herbs*, by Drs. David Frawley and Vasant Lad, (a book to which I contributed) also indicates in great detail the Ayurvedic use of herbs.

A Six-fold Therapeutics

In many Ayurvedic textbooks, you see references to six major forms of therapy mentioned by Charaka:

1. Lightening therapy (*Langhana*) — procedure to decrease body weight and purify the system. In this understanding of therapeutics, Panchakarma is seen as part of lightening therapy.

2. Nourishing Therapy (*Brihana*) — procedure to increase body weight and nourish the system.
3. Drying Therapy (*Rukshana*) — procedure to help reduce fat.
4. Oleation Therapy (*Snehana*) — procedure to promote unctuousness in the body.
5. Fomentation Therapy (*Swedana*) — procedure to induce sweating.
6. Astringent Therapy (*Stambana*) — procedure to reduce the flow of fluids in the body.

Although this system is mentioned in the textbooks, it is seldom incorporated into the regular practice of Ayurveda. Obviously Vata needs nourishing, oleation and possibly fomentation therapy; Kapha needs drying, lightening, fomentation and possibly astringent therapy; and Pitta may need nourishing, drying and astringent therapy — but which specific therapy to emphasize for each dosha, and when and why? Then there is the question of whether Astringent therapy is different from Drying therapy and how so. The answers to these questions remain a little vague in modern day Ayurveda.

Actually these therapies are part of the ancient Ayurveda. When we know how to use the ancient Ayurveda, we will know how to apply these therapies in the most precise way.

Conclusion

Since these first chapters are a summary of modern Ayurveda rather than expositions of the whole science, I won't go into more detail on the basic divisions of medical science: etiology, symptomatology and therapeutics. I will also resist discussing further the major principles within Ayurvedic medicine: doshas, dhatus, malas, agnis and srotas. However, it is my sincere hope that the outline of Ayurveda set forth in these chapters will help clarify what, in some books, tends to be a very complex and even disorganized subject. Without a clear grasp of the essential principles of modern Ayurveda, it will be difficult to grasp its differences from the ancient Ayurveda, which we will explore next.

The Ancient Ayurveda

Glimpses of the ancient Ayurveda are found in the ancient science of the stars known as *Jyotish* or Vedic Astrology. It was commonly understood in the ancient days that medicine and astrology were sister sciences and should always be practiced together. Even Hippocrates, the father of Western medicine, said: "He who does not know the science of the stars is not worthy of calling himself a physician."

If this is the case, then why did Ayurveda and Vedic astrology split off from one another? The answer, in my opinion, is that Vedic astrology lost its way some three to four thousand years ago and became such a distorted system that it was not very useful for making accurate predictions in any of the major fields of living, including health and disease. When Ayurvedic practitioners experienced this fact, they broke away from the proponents of their sister science. This happened not only with Ayurveda, but with many other Vedic disciplines as well. A true astrology is a multi-disciplinary and interdisciplinary tool par excellence; therefore, when Vedic astrology declined, so did all holistic knowledge, and the Vedic disciplines became isolated from one another.

There are great Vedic scholars and pundits who firmly believe that the present day practice of Vedic astrology is accurate, useful and complete. Nevertheless, the ancient Vedic astrology, which I uncovered and used in the process of rediscovering the ancient Ayurveda, has little in common with modern Vedic astrological practice. I believe that the present day practices of Vedic and Western astrology tend not to give accurate or precise predictions in any field of living. Fortunately, the restoration of the ancient Ayurveda and the ability to benefit from it does not require the acceptance of my belief about astrology.

To continue my theory, once Ayurveda separated from Vedic astrology, errors began to creep into Ayurveda. The astrological paradigm of disease emphasized seven major diseases, which corresponded to the seven major planets. Now that it was no longer possible to tell what planet ruled which of the seven primal diseases, Ayurveda began to focus on the specific symptoms of these seven primal diseases and gave disease names to these symptoms. They began to speak of eighty diseases being caused by Vata dosha, forty diseases by Pitta dosha, and twenty diseases by Kapha dosha. This is where, in my opinion, modern Ayurveda began to err, because focusing on the leaves and branches of disease is never as valuable as focusing on the major roots.

When I use the term "modern Ayurveda," I am including Charaka and Sushruta, the founders of modern day Ayurveda. The system I call the "ancient Ayurveda" stems from the pre-Vedic or very early Vedic civilization, before India began to use a caste system based on birth and heredity. That could not have happened while there was a true science of the stars to inform people as to their natural caste tendencies (see Part Three) and to steer society in healthy directions through the promotion of effective caste institutions.

The other error which crept into Ayurveda was the belief that the constitutional nature of the individual most often determined the diseases to which they would be prone. The ancient Ayurveda indicates that one's constitutional type neither determines nor directly influences one's disease tendencies. Let's look at one of the major diseases of the ancient Ayurveda — the disease of dryness. Any constitutional type can have this disease if the planet Saturn governs their physical health, but the likelihood of getting this disease and its severity will be greater for those of a Vata constitution. In treating the disease tendency, the practitioner wants to keep an eye on the constitutional type so as not to unnecessarily aggravate it. That is the extent of the relationship between constitution and disease, according to the ancient Ayurveda.

For these reasons, practitioners of modern day Ayurveda are not always successful in preventing, diagnosing or treating chronic ailments, whereas the ancient model has the capacity for great success in such cases. The public is becoming aware of the discrepancy between the claims of modern Ayurveda and its results — so much so that many individuals (Eastern disciples in particular) no longer go to Ayurvedic practitioners when they are seriously ill. They have lost their confidence in this modern model of Ayurveda. However, modern Ayurveda has much wisdom to be retained when integrated with the ancient system.

The Ancient Ayurveda

We find the basis of the ancient Ayurveda in some of the astrological texts. The text which I find to be the most concise and complete is Maharishi Parasara's *Brihat Parasara Hora Sastra.* Many consider Parasara to be one of the great enlightened sages who helped create the science of astrology through inner cognition. My own view is that he was a compiler and commentator on the more ancient oral traditions of astrology. He often refers to different schools of astrology and their various viewpoints without definitively choosing any one of them. Nevertheless, he is a worthy source of knowledge in this field.

How can I say the ancient science of the stars was lost many thousands of years ago and still quote from sources available today? The basic knowledge from these texts is not incorrect, but I believe certain key principles which allow proper application have been left out. Such keys can and should only be discovered in the depths of one's own awareness. The adage that knowledge is structured in consciousness is true for all disciplines of study, but it is particularly true for astrological science.

What does Parasara say about Ayurveda in relationship to the science of the stars? First, he indicates that each planet is related to a particular humour or group of humours:

Sun = Pitta

Moon = Vata and Kapha

Mars = Pitta

Mercury = Vata, Pitta and Kapha

Jupiter = Kapha

Venus = Kapha and Vata

Saturn = Vata

The North Node of the Moon is deemed to be like Saturn, and the South Node of the Moon is like the North Node and Saturn, although some suggest it is like Mars.

There is some confusion about Mercury governing all three humours. Most commentators think this means Mercury is a tri-doshic planet, whereas I strongly feel that it means Mercury takes on the humoural characteristics of the planet or planets with which it is associated. So if Mercury is associated with Mars, Jupiter and Saturn, Mercury would then be tri-doshic in nature, but only in that circumstance of being associated with three planets.

Next we learn that each planet governs a taste. As we'll see later when we describe a taste, we are also describing the properties of the planet relating to it and the disease tendency of that planet. Parasara also correlates the planets and the tissue elements, which helps our understanding of how particular tastes build particular tissues and lead to certain diseases:

PLANET	TASTE	TISSUE	HUMOUR
Sun	Pungent	Bone	Pitta
Moon	Salty	Blood	Vata/Kapha
Mars	Bitter	Bone Marrow	Pitta
Mercury	Mixed Taste	Lymph	Vata/Pitta/Kapha
Jupiter	Sweet	Adipose or Fat	Kapha
Venus	Sour	Reproductive	Kapha/Vata
Saturn	Astringent	Muscle	Vata

Sweet Taste and the Disease of Heaviness

According to Charaka, sweet taste has a tissue-building (anabolic) wholesome effect on the seven tissue elements in the body. It soothes the mind and senses, gives strength and good complexion, and builds immunity. It alleviates weakness, emaciation, and the ravages of disease or poisoning; relieves fits, fainting, and burning sensations; and promotes healthy skin, hair and voice. It calms Pitta and Vata, and is heavy, cooling and unctuous in its effects. It is generally nourishing, soothing and invigorating.

In excess, it causes the disease symptoms related to excess Kapha: obesity, loss of appetite, nausea, excess phlegm in the stomach, throat and lungs, and excess salivation.

The ancient Ayurveda suggests that sweet taste creates the first major disease tendency: THE DISEASE OF HEAVINESS. This is a Jupiterian disease. In this disease, adipose tissue becomes excessive, with all the related symptoms reflecting excess heaviness. This is a kaphagenic disease. Note that the planet Jupiter has always signified the quality of expansiveness, and the processes of absorption and assimilation. Jupiter signifies inner stability, balance and strength, but it also relates to diseases due to excesses such as gluttony.

R. J. (Denver, CO)

"I went through a phase in my life where I was overweight, melancholic and depressed. I used sweets as a means of trying to cope with my problems. When Ed was able to convince me that my love of sweets was actually a sign of the disease of heaviness, and convinced me to substitute bitter taste for sweet taste as a corrective therapy, I was on the road to recovery."

Sour Taste and the Disease of Oiliness

According to Charaka, sour taste improves the taste of all food and enkindles the digestive fire. It also nourishes and energizes the body (anabolic), helps clear the mind, strengthens the sense organs, nourishes the heart, promotes strength and the alleviation of excess Vata. It helps in moistening and swallowing food as well as in digestion. It is refreshing, unctuous, light and hot.

In excess, sour taste causes thirst, burning sensations in the throat and chest, teeth sensitivity, vitiation of blood tissue, decomposition of muscle tissue, flaccidity, edema in patients who have fallen into any doshic deficiency, and suppuration of wounds. This taste can aggravate Pitta through toxification of the blood and it can liquefy Kapha. Lastly, it can derange the reproductive tissues.

The ancient Ayurveda suggests that sour taste is primarily unctuous and, consequently, the second major disease tendency which relates to this taste and the planet Venus is THE DISEASE OF OILINESS. The body becomes too oily and this affects not only the reproductive system, but also the kidneys and bladder, the organs relating to Venus. Note that the planet Venus relates to the culinary arts and the deliciousness of food. It also relates to the senses and their clarity and strength of functioning.

An interesting issue arises with this disease of oiliness and its relationship to modern Ayurveda. Parasara says that Venus is a planet with a Kapha-Vata doshic nature. Modern day Ayurveda says that oil is the attribute of both Pitta and Kapha. So does sour taste aggravate primarily Kapha and Vata or Kapha and Pitta? Modern Ayurveda definitely states that it aggravates Kapha and Pitta and pacifies Vata, but the ancient Ayurveda states emphatically that sour taste relieves the dryness of Vata. It should only be used for that purpose. Implicit in such a statement is the inference that it aggravates Pitta and Kapha.

In *The Lost Secrets of Ayurvedic Acupuncture*, by Dr. Frank Ros, he definitively states that the kidney-bladder meridians (which relate to Venus) are Vata in nature, and thus we can reason that excess sour taste may aggravate some attributes (other than dryness) of Vata dosha through the kidney and bladder meridians.

J. A. (Santa Fe, NM)

"I was drinking lots of sour teas, such as raspberry and hibiscus, because I enjoyed them. One day I got the world's worst prostate and bladder infection and couldn't figure out why. Then I got another one a few months later that was just as severe. Not wanting to take any more antibiotics, I went to Ed for alternatives, who suggested that I had the disease of oiliness and that sour taste was aggravating my natural disease tendency. I was reluctant to do drying therapy because I had been told my body type was Vata, which makes me too dry, but I eventually tried it and got excellent results — no more infections, and I feel stronger and more capable of fighting off infections. I no longer trust the idea that body type is a major indicator of disease tendency."

Salty Taste and the Disease of Coldness

If you are having trouble reconciling the two models of Ayurveda, this is understandable. Try not to demand such reconciliation. They may be mutually exclusive is some ways, which is very apparent in the discussion of salty taste.

According to Charaka, salty taste is moistening. It helps break up, loosen or dissolve obstructions, but produces stickiness. It serves as a digestive appetizer by promoting salivation, is laxative and carminative, liquifies Kapha, clarifies the channels of circulation, and brings about tenderness to all the bodily organs. Salty taste is neither very heavy, unctuous or hot.

In excess, it causes aggravation of Pitta and blood tissue, thirst, heating sensation, depletion of muscle tissue, erosion, skin problems, obstruction in the functioning of the senses, loss of reproductive capacity and premature wrinkling, graying and baldness. Other commentators have suggested it also causes fluid retention, swelling, and disruption in the electrolyte balance.

The ancient Ayurveda indicates that this taste creates the lunar disease known as THE DISEASE OF COLDNESS. The body is seventy-five percent water and water is very cold. When we are "too salty," we tend to retain too much water in the cells and this brings on the disease of coldness.

The Moon is soft, soothing and gentle like the action of salt. The Moon is also cold. I have shown clients, time and time again, that when they reduce salt intake, they begin recovering from the disease of coldness. Modern Ayurveda would give salt to relieve the coldness of Vata and Kapha, a strategy that never works unless the coldness is due to another disease known as the disease of dryness. (Please reserve judgment about this ancient science in relationship to modern Ayurveda until you read the complete paradigm of each disease in later chapters).

F. S. (Fairfield, IA)

"I was on a special course for the development of consciousness and, at some point, I remembered that my teacher had said that he had not taken salt for long periods of time as part of his spiritual training, so I decided to do the same. It didn't seem like any big deal. This habit stayed with me for a number of years thereafter, and when my health began to fail, I didn't suspect any correlation between my reduction in salt intake and my ailments. I had been told that I was a Pitta body type, so I figured less salt was good for me. Ed convinced me otherwise. Now that I am taking liberal amounts of salt in my diet, my health is improving and I am finally gaining weight again. For a while the food was just going right through me, largely undigested. My small intestine was a mess. Now my whole system has corrected itself with a little help from my friend: salt!"

Pungent Taste and the Disease of Heat

According to Charaka, this taste helps promote the digestion and absorption of food, keeps the mouth clean, helps purify the sense organs, helps clarify the sense of taste, reduces fat and sticky properties in the body, kills germs, breaks up obstructions and blood clots, and reduces Kapha while aggravating Vata and Pitta. It is light, hot and unctuous. Charaka indicates that, in excess, it brings impotency, giddiness or unconsciousness, loss of strength, emaciation, heat and thirst, and mental weakness. It can also bring asthma.

The ancient Ayurveda suggests that this taste brings THE DISEASE OF HEAT. The Sun, the ruler of this taste, has all the qualities of heat.

L. T. (Albuquerque, NM)

"When I moved to the Southwest, I got into the habit of eating a lot of hot, spicy Mexican food. At first it didn't seem to agree with me, but as I ate it more and more, I developed a real liking for it. After a few years I began to have allergies for the first time. I also became prone to flu and fevers. Ed convinced me that spicy taste was aggravating my tendency to the disease of heat. After cutting out this taste in my diet for about two months, I began to notice major relief from my symptoms. Now I don't even like hot, spicy things — I think I was addicted to what was actually harming my body! One Ayurvedic doctor had suggested many years before that I was a Vata body type, which tends to be too cold, and, therefore, I could take a little hot and spicy food as long as it didn't dry me out too much or cause me to become constipated. That may have biased me towards pungent tasting foods and drinks, because I never got constipated from them. I'm much clearer now that body type and disease type are two different things."

Bitter Taste and the Disease of Lightness

According to Charaka, bitter taste is antitoxic and germicidal. It promotes dryness, causes firmness of the skin and muscles. It dispels gas, promotes digestion and relieves Pitta and Kapha, while aggravating Vata due to its depleting effects on the tissues. It is unctuous, cold and light. When used in excess, it depletes the bodily tissues, causes roughness in the circulatory channels, reduces strength, and causes emaciation, weariness, giddiness, dryness of mouth and unconsciousness.

The ancient Ayurveda suggests that this taste leads to THE DISEASE OF LIGHTNESS, primarily a Pitta disease under the influence of the planet Mars. This too is controversial from the perspective of modern Ayurvedic practitioners, since they use bitter taste to relieve Pitta! The ancient Ayurveda would encourage the use of bitters for this disease, but only for purgation. It is an example of using like to treat like, but only in excess form, as when electroshock therapy is used to treat Vata mental derangement. Note that the planet Mars has many of the purificatory qualities of bitter taste. Once again, please reserve judgment until you see the complete disease paradigm and modes of treatment set forth in detail.

J. K. (Chicago, IL)

"All the Ayurvedic people agreed that I am clearly a Pitta body type and thus I was encouraged to take a lot of bitter herbs, both as purgatives and as teas. I started literally to waste away. Ed convinced me that I have a tendency to the disease of lightness and that I should take purgatives only in mild doses and not too frequently. In addition I should never take bitter teas, but only sweet nourishing drinks. I'm doing a lot better now, even though I'm still not totally clear as to all the distinctions between the system of Ayurveda Ed uses and the modern system."

Astringent Taste and the Disease of Dryness

According to Charaka, astringent taste sedates and constipates. It produces pressure on the affected part, causing stiffness and granulation. It alleviates Kapha and stems the flow of blood. It absorbs body fluid and is dry, cold and heavy. In excess, it causes emaciation, dry mouth, heart trouble, distention of the abdomen, constriction of circulation, darkening of the complexion (aggravated Vata) and impotency, constipation, obstructed flatus, weariness, thirst, and stiffness.

The ancient Ayurveda suggests that this taste leads to THE DISEASE OF DRYNESS, ruled by Saturn. Saturn is dry, cold and constricting.

S. S. (Colorado Springs, Co)

"I am definitely a Kapha type when it comes to constitutional typing. Therefore, astringent taste should be good for me and help reduce my blood pressure. Wrong! It didn't work. It actually seemed to increase my blood pressure! Then along comes Ed and he predicts that astringent taste will actually cause this problem in a person with the disease of dryness. It blew my mind! So then he gave me this herb formula which was sour tasting and it also aggravated me until I reduced the amount and strength of it. Now I seem to be doing a lot better."

NOTE: Sometimes people react too strongly to a medicine at first. Or when they find out what is supposedly good for them, they may go overboard in treating themselves. Part of health education is teaching someone that a good, natural medicine need not be taken in large or frequent doses. It's enough to start changing the predominant taste from a bad one to a good one and let the disease tendency and nature take care of the rest.

Mixed Taste and the Mixed Type of Disease

The ancient Ayurveda includes a seventh disease category. When Mercury governs physical health, then Mercury takes on the disease or diseases of the planets with which it is associated. This type of disease is difficult to diagnose and treat precisely because it often is a mixture of different disease tendencies. It is also possible for Mercury not to be associated with any other planet, in which case it takes on its own characteristics through the meridians related to it. This is why the ancient teachers thought that a physician needed to be an excellent astrologer as well.

If Mercury is associated with Venus, then the meridians related to Mercury as well as Venus will show tendencies of the disease of oiliness. Fortunately, only this disease-type is convoluted; the others are more straightforward. With the Mercurial disease, one must be careful to treat the symptoms as they appear.

A. D. (Denver, CO)

> "It was explained to me by Ed that I need to avoid both salty and astringent tastes and instead use more pungent and sour tastes. It seems to work. I no longer suffer from the dryness and cold like I used to and I think I understand why. I say 'I think I understand,' because this mixed disease-type seems to be somewhat complicated, but as long as it works, I'm happy."

Confirmation of the Ancient Ayurveda

Can we find any reference to this ancient Ayurvedic approach in the modern Ayurvedic literature? In Chapter XXVI of the *Charaka Samhita*, Charaka talks of the great debates among various sages about the science of taste and how his "enlightened group" definitively settles all of these disputes. One of the sages, Varyovida, whose approach Charaka does not embrace, suggests that there are six tastes: heavy, light, cold, hot, unctuous and non-unctuous. In my judgment this sage was a late representative of the ancient Ayurveda.

Another sage mentioned by Charaka is Sakunteya Brahmana. He states that there are just two tastes: nourishing and emaciating. This is also accepted by the ancient Ayurveda. Three planets are benefic in nature: Jupiter, Venus and the Moon. One of the meanings of "benefic" is "that which is anabolic or building and nourishing in effect." These three planets signify the three anabolic diseases: heaviness, oiliness and coldness. Three other planets are malefic in nature: Sun, Mars and Saturn. One of the meanings of "malefic" is "that which is catabolic or purifying in nature." These three planets signify the three catabolic diseases: heat, lightness and dryness. Thus, it is not an over-generalization to suggest that catabolic types need nourishing taste and therapy and anabolic types need purifying and emaciating taste.

Charaka mentions a third sage, Purnaksa Maudgalya, who says there are three tastes: nourishing, emaciating, and having both of these properties. It appears that he is including the mixed-type of disease as the third taste.

V. S.. (Fairfield, IA)

"In my health consultation, Ed suggested that my disease type is ruled by Saturn, and that in addition to oleation therapy in all its many forms, I need to include more protein in my diet and less carbohydrates and fat. When I do this, I notice an immediate surge in energy. Now, when I eat out and don't get enough protein, I know that I will suffer an energy lag soon after. I've even begun taking protein powder with me on trips so that I can 'doctor' my meals when needed."

C. S. (Milwaukee, WI)

"I have what Ed calls 'the Jupiter disease tendency.' Thus, I'm on a lightening therapy program. No, I don't have to stand out under a tree in a thunderstorm. Lightening therapy means any routine or therapeutics which brings lightness to the body and increases catabolism. In addition, I take in less protein as compared to carbohydrates and fats. It seems to work well for me! I no longer suffer from the heaviness and fatigue which used to so debilitate me — at least as long as I stay away from the sweets!"

Further Correlation

The seven major disease types within the ancient Ayurveda are: 1) the disease of heat ruled by the Sun; 2) its opposite, the disease of coldness ruled by the Moon; 3) the disease of lightness, ruled by Mars; 4) its opposite, the disease of heaviness, ruled by Jupiter; 5) the disease of dryness, ruled by Saturn; 6) its opposite, the disease of oiliness, ruled by Venus; and 7) a mixed type of disease, ruled by Mercury. All other disease names are nothing but symptoms of these seven major disease types, and to know our own disease type and how to prevent or treat it is I feel the most valuable knowledge we can ever acquire. We may know everything about our constitution and how to treat it and still be in ill-health without this knowledge which comes from the ancient Ayurveda.

These seven diseases are treated with the seven therapies we have already mentioned: heating, cooling, lightening, nourishing, drying, oleating and mixed type of treatment. These treatments can be conducted allopathically (treating like with unlike) or homeopathically (treating like with like). The relationship between the disease types and various modes of treatment is set forth in the following table. Note that the allopathic therapy relates to the disease opposite it, i.e. fomentation therapy is for the disease of coldness and cooling therapy is for the disease of heat. Also note the importance of metals in the ancient Ayurveda and their use in homeopathy:

PRIMAL DISEASE THERAPY	ALLOPATHIC THERAPY (including taste)	HOMEOPATHIC
Heat	Fomentation (pungent)	Homeopathic Gold
Cold	Cooling (salty)	Homeopathic Silver
Lightness	Lightening (bitter)	Homeopathic Iron
Heaviness	Nourishing (sweet)	Homeopathic Tin
Dryness	Drying (astringent)	Homeopathic Lead
Oiliness	Oleation (sour)	Homeopathic Copper
Mixed	One or more of the above	Homeopathic Mercury

The next table sets forth how the various organs systems and meridians of Chinese medicine relate to the seven planets and their disease tendencies. This may surprise those who are used to thinking of Chinese medicine as a totally separate system from the Ayurvedic one.

PLANET & DISEASE	CHINESE MERIDIANS
Sun and Heat	Small Intestine and Heart
Moon and Coldness	Triple Warmer and Pericardium
Mars and Lightness	Gall Bladder and Governer Vessel
Jupiter and Heaviness	Conception Vessel and Liver
Saturn and Dryness	Stomach and Spleen
Venus and Oiliness	Bladder and Kidney

It is important to understand these correlations because, when we treat a particular disease tendency, one of the basic modes of treatment will be to treat the related meridians. The first meridian listed is always the more surface meridian; the second is the deeper of the two. When the deeper organ and meridian is affected, it is a more serious problem than when the surface organ is affected. For example, bladder problems are generally not as serious as kidney problems. The large intestine is more easily treated than the lung, etc.

Some may wonder why the two Vessels, Conception and Governor, are assigned respectively to Jupiter and Mars. A study of the significations of the two planets, and the functioning of the two vessels should provide a satisfactory answer. Jupiter signifies the conception of children and Mars the ability to use the will skillfully in governing one's life. The healthy functioning of these two vessels insures a normal ability to conceive children and manage one's life. Some of the other designations between planets and organs are ancient and non-controversial among true esotericists: Mercury/lungs, Jupiter/liver, Mars/gall bladder, Sun/heart, Venus/kidney, and Saturn/spleen. Since the surface organs clearly go with the deep ones, it is equally proper to designate the Sun with the small intestine, Venus with the bladder, Saturn with the stomach and Mercury with the large intestine.

The triple warmer and pericardium meridians (sometimes called Circulation/Sex Meridian) are special cases which can be seen clearly to correlate with the Moon once a study has been made of Chinese medicine and its relationship to both Ayurveda and the science of the stars. The purpose of this book is not to prove this ancient system (proof of such a system is beyond the capacity of any one person), but to elaborate it in detail.

The following table sets forth the relationship between the planets and their disease tendencies and the endocrine system. When we think about a particular primal disease, we should also be thinking of its dhatu, meridians, and hormonal system. These will be the most

PLANET & DISEASE	HORMONAL SYSTEM
Sun and Heat	Pineal Gland
Moon and Coldness	Thymus
Mars and Lightness	Adrenals and Pancreas
Jupiter and Heaviness	Gonads (Testes/Ovaries)
Saturn and Dryness	Prostate/Cervix
Venus and Oiliness	Thyroid and Parathyroid
Mercury and Mixed Type	Pituitary

controversial designations of all, largely because the endocrine system remains somewhat of a mystery even to Western scientists.

To summarize: in analyzing the disease of heat we would want to focus on a person's bone tissue, small intestine and heart meridians, and the pineal gland in terms of treatment. The same would hold true for diagnostics. When trying to determine the disease tendency of the person, we would have to consider the above three factors, particularly when considering the disease of heat. How to do this most effectively is explored in Part Two of this book.

In treating a primal disease, we would use the particular therapy which relates to the particular disease in question, either allopathically and/or homeopathically. How to do so most effectively is explored in Part Three of this book.

The Two Systems Compared

Etiology

I have already indicated that any medical science, including Ayurveda, is fundamentally the study of the etiology of disease, and its symptomatology and therapeutics. In Chapter 2, I presented a comprehensive understanding of the causes of disease, the six stages of the disease process, and the three pathways through which disease travels. Modern Ayurveda and the ancient Ayurveda both accept all these distinctions, so there are no major differences in this arena.

Symptomatology

Chapter 2 contained an introduction to symptomatology. Part Two of this book thoroughly discusses the various symptoms of each of the seven primal diseases. Notice a different emphasis in exploring symptomatology. Modern Ayurveda groups symptoms around the three doshas or the specific disease in question: eighty Vata diseases, forty Pitta diseases, and twenty Kapha diseases. The ancient Ayurveda suggests that the modern day Ayurvedic diagnosis and treatment of the doshas is too spread out, and groups symptoms around the seven primal diseases. All these symptoms can be related to the three doshas, since the planet governing each disease has its own doshic make-up, but the disease type dominates.

A Solar Pitta disease has different symptoms from a Martian Pitta disease. One predominantly causes symptoms of heat; the other causes more symptoms of lightness. The same holds true for Kapha diseases. A Jupiterian Kapha disease is different from a Venusian or Lunar one (heaviness versus oiliness versus coldness). A Saturn disease emphasizes the dryness of Vata, a Lunar disease emphasizes the coldness of both Vata and Kapha.

Therapeutics

Although the ancient Ayurveda accepts all the same kinds of therapeutics as modern Ayurveda, it uses the seven major therapeutics — fomentation, cooling, nourishing, lightening, drying, oiling and mixed — in more precise ways. Its practitioners can know which attribute of Vata, Pitta or Kapha to treat, and how to do so most effectively.

Many of the preliminary procedures in modern Ayurveda's use of Panchakarma, as practiced by some organizations, such as taking oil and ghee both internally and externally to "loosen the ama," is contra-indicated for someone with the disease of oiliness. Giving fomentation to someone with the disease of heat or giving lightening therapy to the person with lightheadedness is also not advised.

If we were to go to India today, we would find that Ayurveda and modern Western homeopathy are treated as two different medical sciences. Modern Ayurvedic practitioners rely on dietetics and herbs and few venture into the field of homeopathy, but the ancient Ayurveda always used both allopathy and homeopathy together.

How ancient Ayurveda uses the science of taste is obviously quite different from modern Ayurveda. Modern Ayurveda uses salty taste to relieve Vata and Kapha, both of which share the attribute of cold; ancient Ayurveda uses avoidance of salty taste to treat the disease of coldness. Modern Ayurveda uses bitter taste to treat Pitta. Ancient Ayurveda suggest that bitter taste aggravates those suffering from the Pitta disease of lightness, except when used as a purgative. The use of the other tastes are compatible in both systems, except that ancient Ayurveda leaves open the possibility that the Kidney-Bladder meridians and the Vata meridians, according to Dr. Frank Ros, are still aggravated through sour taste.

Certainly, the eight clinical disciplines remain the same in both the ancient and modern Ayurveda: Internal Medicine, Pediatrics, Diseases of the Eye, Ear, Nose and Throat, Psychiatry, Surgery, Toxicology, Rejuvenation and Virilization.

Doshas And Constitution

Ancient and modern Ayurveda agree as to the number of doshas and their basic qualities, but part company on the relationship of physiological constitution to disease tendency. Modern Ayurveda believes that if a person's constitution is being treated, the practitioner is doing the maximum to ensure the person doesn't become diseased. Modern Ayurveda theory admits the distinction between prakruti (constitution) and vikruti (present doshic balance regardless of one's constitutional type), but believes that most often vikruti will follow the tendency created from prakruti.

The ancient Ayurveda is interested in constitution, but believes it to be a secondary consideration for health and longevity. Ancient Ayurveda suggests that one's major disease tendency is not directly related to constitution, but that a person's constitution can indirectly affect the major disease tendency in terms of it severity and likelihood of manifestation. An individual with a Vata constitution is more likely to manifest a severe disease of dryness than someone with a Pitta or Kapha constitution.

The ancient Ayurveda accepts the five types of Vata, Pitta and Kapha established in the modern Ayurveda. There are no significant differences between the two systems in respect to this topic. It also uses the same twenty attributes for describing the qualities and functioning of each dosha, but it is able to isolate certain key attributes in relationship to the science of taste and the diseases related to the excess use of that taste. Thus, it is not enough to know if Vata is deranged; one must also know which attribute of Vata is the primary one causing the disease.

L. M. (Albuquerque, NM)

"I am a predominantly Kapha and Pitta body type and thus I could never understand why I suffered from nagging problems of dryness and constipation throughout my whole life. When Ed explained that I have a tendency to the disease of dryness, even though that tendency is somewhat mitigated by my body type, it made perfect sense to me, and now I treat myself quite differently than before. I worry about my disease type first and constitution only secondarily. This understanding of how to distinguish one's disease tendency from one's constitutional type has made all the difference in the world in how I handle my own health-care."

T. D. (Fairfield, IA)

"I've always been told by the Ayurvedic experts that I am predominantly Vata Dosha in my constitutional makeup, but I never had much success dealing with my ailments through treating Vata. When Ed suggested that my disease tendency was that of heat, and then suggested that I use cooling therapies for treating this problem, I was a little scared. Just imagine: I'm told to use over long periods of time the very therapy which supposedly aggravates my constitutional type and brings poor health. But I did it and the results were excellent!

What I like about Ed's work is that he doesn't tell you what to do. He merely suggests a possible blueprint for dealing with one's own unique health issues, and he explains this blueprint in enough depth that one can decide for oneself its value and what parts of it to accept or reject. It is true health education. But, at the same time, it may only be appropriate for those individuals who are confident enough to treat themselves once they have had the proper health education."

Dhatus

The ancient Ayurveda accepts the seven dhatus in the same way modern Ayurveda does, but it pinpoints the importance of one particular dhatu for each primal disease: the disease of heat and bone tissue, the disease of cold and blood tissue, the disease of lightness and marrow tissue, the disease of heaviness and fat tissue, the disease of dryness and muscle tissue, the disease of oiliness and reproductive tissue, and the mixed type of disease and lymph tissue. Modern Ayurvedic practitioners are good at theorizing about the dhatus, but perhaps not as adept at using this knowledge in practical therapeutics.

A. K. (Milwaukee, WI)

"When I used to go to alternative practitioners, I was told some useful things and some off-base things, but never that my lymph system was bad. Then I got lymph cancer. After a protracted battle, I finally got better. So imagine my surprise when Ed suggested, as part of a health reading and without any input from me, that I would have a tendency to the mixed-type of disease ruled by Mercury and lymph disorders. Now I no longer worry about this problem because I can clearly see the causes, symptoms, and preventive treatment for this problem. This is health education at its best."

Malas

Both schools of Ayurveda use the malas in similar ways, except the ancient model ties one particular attribute and its corresponding symptomatology to each waste product. For example, one can indicate that the symptoms related to urine production and flow are due to the disease of Pitta, but one can also indicate that the symptoms relate to both the disease of heat and lightness. This symptomatology is more precise than the modern one, because it distinguishes two different types of primal Pitta diseases and offers different modes of treatment for each. The same holds true for Vata and Kapha doshas. (Note: Vata relates to feces and Kapha to sweat)

R. J. (Austin, TX)

"I was told that my constipation was due to problems with Vata dosha and dryness, and to take in a lot more oily substances. This worked to some degree, but not fully. Then Ed explained that I had a tendency to the disease of coldness and that warmth was the essential attribute needed to treat the constipation. It worked — and far better than taking in oil. Now I see where it is not enough to treat a particular dosha. You must also know the attribute of that dosha which is most out of balance."

Agnis

The understanding of the various agnis is the same with both approaches to Ayurveda, but the treatment may be very different. A modern-day practitioner may note variable Agni in a Vata person and want to give salt as a remedy. A practitioner of the ancient school would not do this if he saw the person suffered from the disease of coldness. A modern practitioner might feel agni was too high and give bitters for it; a practitioner of ancient Ayurveda would not do this if the disease of lightness was diagnosed.

J. K. (Philadelphia, PA)

> "I was told to take bitters for low agni. It made things worse! It ends up that I actually suffered from bile accumulation in the stomach due to the disease of lightness, and that this is different from low agni. It was nourishing, sweet tasting foods and herbs which eventually improved my digestion, not bitters. I must admit that I wasn't very confident in what Ed said. It went against my whole Ayurvedic training. Now I realize that the Ayurveda I was taught was not the whole picture."

Srotas

Both systems use the sixteen srotas: Seven srotas relate to the seven dhatus, three to the malas, and two relate to the female system (both of which are important in both systems of Ayurveda). The same can be said for the mind channel. The first three srotas — Pranavaha Srotas, Annavaha Srotas and Udakvaha Srotas — are subsumed by the ancient Ayurveda under the fourteen more specific meridians of Chinese medicine. Modern Ayurveda has no systematic way of integrating the meridians into its framework, nor have its theoreticians tried to do so.

K. E. (Denver, CO)

"Every time I would go to a chiropractor, they would muscle-test me and find some energy imbalance in some new organ. First it was my liver that was the problem, then the kidneys, then the spleen. I think I went through the whole gamut. Finally, Ed explained that I suffered from the disease of heaviness and that the liver and conceptions were the prime culprits. Any other organ imbalance would be merely a symptom of the underlying disruptions in these two meridians. I began to study these two meridians and their related points carefully. Then I studied different methods for treating both the points and the meridians. Now I am in very good health through treating these regularly and also doing lightening therapy. Ed's understanding of how to correlate health problems and meridian systems is quite amazing."

Case Study

B. was on crutches because of a severe pain on the inside of his foot, which no one seemed to be able to diagnose or treat effectively. It soon became apparent to me that he had the disease of oiliness and that his pain was exactly on the kidney meridian line of the foot (the kidney and/or bladder are most often affected in this particular disease tendency). He was prescribed drying therapy in all forms. Unfortunately, this gentleman was seeing so many different doctors and therapists at the time that my diagnosis got lost in the shuffle and I never had the chance to do any follow-up with him. This is not uncommon. Many people who have grown up with Western medicine find a model such as presented in this book too simplistic. They just can't accept the idea that "oiliness," for example, is the root cause of their ill-health.

The Endocrine System

The ancient Ayurveda had an understanding of the endocrine system in relation to the seven primal diseases and I have tried to set this forth in a clear way, although I suggest to people that this aspect of the work should not be taken with the same degree of confidence as the rest of the knowledge. We still have a lot to learn about the endocrine system and its relationship to disease. Modern Ayurveda touches upon this subject but, perhaps, could be organized in a more effective way.

Conclusion

There are many points in common between the two systems of Ayurveda, but there are also major differences, especially in the end result. I believe the practice of modern Ayurveda may be harmful, in many cases, when not tempered with the knowledge of the ancient Ayurveda.

B. C., Holistic Counselor and
Nutritionist (Fairfield, IA)

"I am blessed with moderately good health. However, my 25-year quest for ideal fitness, natural beauty and longevity has elicited a barrage of alternative health-care experiences which span the dozens of choices available in the marketplace. While I'm convinced these natural healing practices offer great promise, their major drawback is a universal, one-size-fits-all mentality.

"Although marketplace Ayurveda made an attempt to determine my particular body type, its classic paradigm of Vata-Pitta-Kapha wasn't nearly precise enough to provide a clear diagnosis. This flaw became extremely apparent to me when I was exposed to Ed's work with the ancient Ayurvedic model. Finally, everything made perfect sense. My symptoms were not random, unrelated imbalances requiring often conflicting therapies, but rather they fit the exact profile of the disease of coldness. By applying the suggested therapeutics derived from this more ancient system of Ayurveda, my digestive weakness, menstrual irregularities and severe chest colds were ameliorated."

PART TWO

Symptomatology and Therapeutics in the Ancient Ayurveda

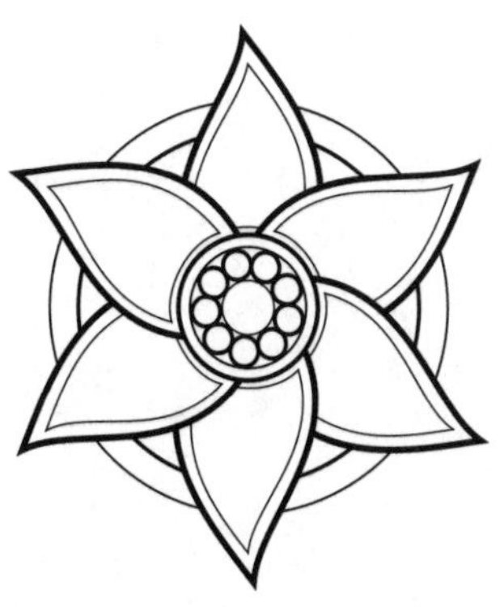

SYMPTOMATOLOGY OF DISEASE

It is quite a challenge to describe all the major symptoms of each primal disease tendency. If it is too elaborate, like some of the homeopathic texts, it becomes too technical. If it is not elaborate enough, it can be of no use to practitioners. I have decided to use the classic eight-fold examination of pulse, urine, feces, skin, eyes, tongue, face and voice, plus four other criteria: the dhatu, two organs, meridians, and the endocrine system related to the disease in question. Voice is an important means for discovering mental symptoms of a particular disease tendency. Urine, feces and skin (including sweat) are, of course, the three malas or waste products. Pulse, tongue, eye and facial diagnosis are very crucial as well. There will also be a miscellaneous category for any other symptoms, if any, which don't conveniently fit within the previous twelve.

Please be alert to the fact that a planet and its disease relate to one or more primary humours, but the focus is more particular: one attribute, i.e. hot or cold, one body tissue, two organ systems, and one endocrine system. Thus, many of the symptoms for the two Pitta planets — Sun and Mars; the three Vata planets, — Saturn, the Moon (Vata and Kapha), and Mercury when not associated with any other planet(s); and the three Kapha planets — Jupiter, Venus and the Moon (Kapha and Vata) — sound alike, but they have a predominant application to different dhatus, organ systems and endocrine systems. Please note that many symptoms are somewhat subjective in nature. We have to utilize our intuition to understand and apply these categories.

The Disease of Heat

PULSE: Wiry, rapid, harsh, nodular and taut, like a jumping frog which is exerting too much energy. The pulse is too hot and volcanic. The small intestine and heart meridian pulses are particularly strong in heat and uplift. These pulses will feel hot and light, but heat will prevail over lightness when compared to the Mars pulse, which exists in a disease of lightness. The pulse may also feel feeble or irregular in some cases of deficiency.

URINE: Scalding or hot, either clear or turbid with thick sediment. The color is yellow to reddish. There may be painful retention.

FECES: Constipation with stools hard and knotty, or with loose stool, particularly in the early morning or evening. The stool may have a yellowish, greenish or red tinge (blood-stained).

SKIN: Sweats too easily and profusely, or, in some cases, the inability to sweat even on exertion in chronic cases. Skin is soft and glistening and may appear ruddy.

TONGUE: Red and sometimes swollen, particularly in the areas of the tongue relating to the small intestine and heart. There can be great thirst or very little thirst in chronic cases.

VOICE: Heated, angry words, or ones which are quite sharp and to the point.

EYES: Vision is defective. The whites of eyes are reddish or yellowish. The person has photophobia. The eyes and/or bones around the eyes are inflamed, tense or sore. The pain appears to move from without inward.

FACE: Appears fierce, tense and often ruddy. Often the nose is unduly red or swollen, with veins showing. Since heat rises, often the neck or forehead is quite hot.

BONE TISSUE: Osteoporosis often accompanied with calcium deficiency, especially in women. The person's physical balance becomes compromised as she gets older, when compared to others her age.

SMALL INTESTINE MERIDIAN: Food passes too quickly through the small intestine with poor assimilation of food. The person may be emaciated. There may be mastitis or tinnitus. The person will be susceptible to high fevers and tropical diseases like malaria. There can be stiff neck, low back pain, night sweats, and headache with a piercing pain in the head or pain in the back of the shoulder. Agni will be too high with excess bile formation.

HEART: Arteriosclerosis, including all types of heart disorders, such as angina, heart palpitation, low or high blood pressure, poor circulation, heart attack, with related symptoms including depression, self-condemnation and sense of worthlessness. The person cannot do things fast enough and is hyper-sensitive to noise and excitement. He may suffer from asthma.

ENDOCRINE SYSTEM: A malfunctioning pineal gland. The pineal gland is definitely related to the Sun and adequate sunlight for regulation of the basic biorhythms of the body, especially sleep patterns.

The pineal gland is not well understood in modern day Western medicine. It is difficult to find books which give symptoms of a malfunctioning pineal gland, and even these books should be viewed with a degree of healthy skepticism.

MISCELLANEOUS: Memory loss, vertigo, deterioration in body fluids, sleeplessness, particularly around midnight. In ancient times, certain forms of cutaneous abnormalities like leprosy were related to the Sun and the disease of heat. The same holds true for epilepsy. The ancient sages also related this solar disease to the incidence of burns, danger from weapons, poison and all types of authority figures.

Serpent deities, being under the influence of the Nodes of the Moon (which eclipse the Sun), were thought of as bringing wrath to a person governed physically by the Sun. The ruling family deity could also bring down wrath if displeased. I mention these things because I believe there is a relationship between the physical body and other more subtle influences, even though Western medical science has some difficulty with such a concept.

Additional Comments:

- Someone with the disease of heat does not always immediately relate to this disease type, because, due to their tendency to poor circulation, they sometimes feel cold in winter or cool weather. Of course, they will also feel quite hot in summer or warm weather due to the same poor circulation.
- Someone who has studied modern Ayurveda will assume that a major symptom of this disease, since it is a Pitta disease, will be high blood pressure. It is more common to have low blood pressure with this disease because of the absence of normal amounts of salt and, thus, water in the system.
- When someone has this, or any of the other six physiological imbalances, they may crave the very taste that puts them the most out of balance — just as an alcoholic craves more alcohol. Thus, to crave pungent taste could be an indication of this disease type.
- Anytime one sees a malabsorption syndrome, which is due to too much heat in the small intestine, then consider this disease paradigm as the cause.

Notice that often the symptomatology is quite paradoxical with the manifestation of symptoms, which are opposite from one case to another, such as extreme constipation to very loose stools. Some of these contrasts in symptoms can be explained through variations in constitution and some through the concept of excess and deficiency, but this would make our discussion of the subject unduly complex and I leave such further elaboration to your reflection.

L. M. (Boulder, CO)

"Ed knew about my heart problems before I could even mention them to him. It sort of shook me up. But after he explained how he knew of this tendency, and the reasons for it, I felt more comfortable. Eventually I was quite grateful for the blueprint he provided me for dealing with this disease, especially since one of his major recommendations — more salt — was contraindicated according to others. The other thing I liked was that he didn't discourage me from working with other health professionals, including Western medical doctors. He kept telling me: 'Just pay attention to the blueprint I give you, and then you decide who else to see and what to follow.' I like this approach. It made me feel self-sufficient."

Case Study

M. came to me complaining of tiredness, fatigue, poor memory and lack of interest in life. She had been practicing Transcendental Meditation™ for a long time, including long courses where one combines fasting and long periods of meditation. She had been examined by doctors trained in Maharishi Ayurveda and had been told that her body type was primarily Vata and secondarily Pitta. For most of the year, she would treat Vata dosha, since this doshic aggravation seemed to best explain her symptoms.

Actually, this lady suffered from the disease of heat ruled by the Sun. She had very low blood pressure, so low that I am surprised others had not tried to address that issue directly. After giving her a whole program for treating the disease of heat, including liberal amounts of sea salt in the diet and a ban on hot, spicy Indian food, she began to feel much better. Now she is an active person with enough energy reserves to carry on her normal responsibilities.

The Disease of Coldness

PULSE: cold, sluggish, receding, vanishing, and feeble. If the basic constitution is more Vata in nature, the pulse may also be somewhat crooked, hollow, and slippery like a snake. If the constitution is more Kapha, the pulse may also be somewhat fleshy, straight, and mildly forceful, like a swan moving over a gentle wave in the water. The pulse may also be irregular and intermittent.

Note: Pulse characteristics are a combination of constitutional typing and doshic imbalances. These characteristics will be particularly noticeable with the triple-warmer (tri-doshic pulse) and pericardium pulses, ruled by the Moon.

URINE: Frequent, profuse, turbid, with sweet odor and more salty in taste than usual. Or the urine may be scanty and dark if vata is more affected. If sweets are taken, there is increased urination. Generally, the urine feels cold, as does the person while urinating.

FECES: Flatulent, with mucus (Kapha) or sometimes with small dry stool and constipation (Vata). Urge to evacuate is present, but the peristalsis is weak, at times, due to coldness.

SKIN: Too little perspiration when cold, too much when hot. Skin can be withered and dried-up. The skin can be very white and milky, or discolored. Scabies, urticaria, and edema may exist.

TONGUE: Prominent papillae, tip is red and painful, excess white mucus on tongue. There may be teeth marks on edges of tongue due to poor agni. There can be a strong desire for sweets.

VOICE: Slow, hoarse, or heavily emotionally-laden speech, or speaking in a hurry (reaction to an inner feeling of time passing too slowly). There is a melancholy mode of expression, or person can't remember what he or she wants to say. In advanced cases there may be slurred speech (and loss of balance) due to degeneration of the cerebellum.

Note: the Moon governs the brain.

EYES: Spots or floaters in the visual field, and poor eyesight in general compared to one's peers. There may be an aching, tired feeling in the eyes, which goes away when the eyes are closed or pressed. It is hard to keep the eyes fixed steadily on some object. There may be photophobia in an overly warm room (opposing factors cause reaction — cold reacts to heat).

FACE: Appears to be too white and cold. Emotional disturbances cause the onset of headaches with chills and trembling.

BLOOD TISSUE: The acid-alkaline balance in the blood is easily upset. The blood becomes too cold, causing lack of vitality and difficulty moving in the morning until one warms up, like a cold snake on a rock waiting for the sun to come up. The liquid, salty, nourishing aspect of the blood becomes too predominant.

Note: the warming aspect of the blood is ruled by Mars through the bone marrow and the hemoglobin produced from the marrow.

TRIPLE-WARMER MERIDIAN: Acute fevers which promote the release of cold and phlegm from the system, headache, "stiffness" of the tongue (slurring), sudden hoarseness, tinnitus, common colds, tonsillitis, pleurisy, and vertigo.

PERICARDIUM MERIDIAN: diarrhea, dysentery, heart and chest pain, stomach-ache, irregular menstruation, scabies and damp skin diseases, especially of the upper extremities. There may be stiffness of tongue, swellings and mental disorders. There can be a strong feeling of suffocation in the chest or weight on the chest in advanced cases. There can also be pain in the hypochondriac region.

ENDOCRINE SYSTEM: The Moon rules the thymus gland, which, according to one school, is often not active in adults, but, according to another school, is responsible for weakened defenses against disease for both children and adults. It can be stimulated throughout life in order to slow the tendency of the thymus gland to degenerate with advancing age. The degeneration of the thymus gland is often related to the impaired functioning of the pericardium meridian. Some feel that the thymus gland activates the T-cells which provide immunity. It is also considered to be a link between the mind and body; positive emotions (the Moon) can promote thymus activity.

MISCELLANEOUS: Gradual drying up of the articulations and their component elements — bones, cartilage, ligaments and blood vessels. There can be alteration in the timbre of the voice or loss of voice when sick. There can be profuse and easy expectoration in the morning upon getting up, writer's cramp, and uterine disease (Moon governs uterus). According to the ancient sages of astrology the Moon brings an increase of sleep and inertia, poor agni, blood poisoning, anemia, and sorrow from the spouse.

Additional Comments:

- Since the Moon is cold, slow or low agni is the primary root of most of the imbalances listed above. One must balance the agni in individuals having this disease tendency.
- The Moon also governs menstruation, pregnancy and lactation, and one must treat the disease of coldness to satisfactorily remedy many female complaints.
- Women often are bothered psychologically by cellulite deposits. In the case of lunar types, this toxic fat deposit is caused by impaired digestion due to low agni and must be treated accordingly.

D. G. (Fairfield, IA)

"I am predominantly Pitta and secondarily Vata dosha and always assumed, based upon my Ayurvedic health consultations, that my health problems were primarily Pitta-related. This puzzled me because the one time I was quite sick for a week or two, I had an abnormally low body temperature and no appetite. Along comes Ed and explains that I have the disease of coldness, with the low agni which often accompanies this disease! Now I know how to treat myself, and although I've had a reoccurrence of the digestive crisis which accompanies this disease paradigm, it only happened when I slipped from Ed's guidelines."

CASE STUDY

G. complained of heavy chest pressure, unbearable at times, along with menstrual difficulties and poor digestion. She was receiving little relief from using classic Ayurveda and Western medicine. It became immediately apparent that she had the disease of coldness, which was being aggravated by living in the cold North. She was advised to move to a warmer climate and to engage in various forms of fomentation therapy. She is doing much better now.

The Disease of Lightness

PULSE: Similar to the quality and style of pulse displayed in the disease of heat, but with more of a light jumpy quality, particularly in the place on the wrist where one finds the gall bladder pulse. The pulse may be more rapid than the heated pulse. It can also appear full, but soft and yielding. There can be skipping of beats. In deficiency, the pulse will appear small and weak.

Note: The Ayurvedic and Tibetan traditions locate the gall bladder pulse on the patient's right hand (middle, surface position), whereas some of the schools of Chinese medicine place it on the left hand (middle surface position).

URINE: There can be a tickling sensation in the urethra extending to the bladder. The consistency of the urine will tend to be clear and light. It is yellow to reddish in color. In advanced cases, there can be involuntary passing of urine.

FECES: Loose with undigested foodstuff, especially if the gallbladder is inflamed and tender. This can alternate with constipation. Both conditions are due to improper release of bile — too much with loose stool and too little with constipation. There can also be cramping pain in or prolapse of the rectum, along with backache.

SKIN: Pallor alternating with a flushed look, cold extremities, with pitting of the skin on pressure. The skin may also be extremely sensitive, with allergic reactions and great sensitivity to touch.

TONGUE: There may be little or no coating on the tongue due to excess agni. The tongue may appear red. There will be excessive appetite and a requirement of inordinately frequent meals followed, at times, by poor digestion due to too much bile.

VOICE: Impatient, hurried, tense, anxious, can't do things fast enough. Becomes excited by the slightest opposition.

EYES: Photophobia, dull red color, but with a sharp, quick, light, penetrating look.

FACE: Pallor until pain, emotion or exertion is experienced, then one can become flushed and fiery-red in complexion.

BONE MARROW TISSUE: A tendency to produce too many red blood cells and iron, resulting in various conditions (hemosiderosis and hemochromatosis) which can all be categorized as iron overload. This overload is deposited in various places in the body, causing many seemingly unrelated symptoms. There can also be various forms of anemia.

GALLBLADDER MERIDIAN: Febrile diseases such as malaria, pain in the hypochondria, rigidity in the neck, diarrhea, excessive hunger, bitter taste in mouth, irregular menstruation, headaches, nosebleed or other forms of excessive bleeding, eye redness, conjunctivitis, and other Pitta symptoms.

GOVERNOR VESSEL: A broad range of symptoms covering all organ systems in the body and their proper maintenance (governing function).

ENDOCRINE SYSTEM: Western medicine has given disease names to various types of hyper- and hypo-functioning of the adrenal glands, i.e. Addison's disease or Cushing's syndrome. People who psychologically or physically push themselves too hard (Mars) can tax the adrenals. "Type-A" behavior is a classic cause and symptom of the disease of lightness.

MISCELLANEOUS: Voracious appetite or absolute loss of appetite, heat and burning in the stomach (gastritis or ulcers), tendency to abortion, lumbago, and pain between the shoulder blades.

The ancient sages suggested that this disease of Mars indicated thirst, high blood pressure, fever due to the accumulation of bile, diseases caused by heat, poison, burns or weapons, epilepsy, and fear from destructive spirits, enemies and robbers. There can also be quarrels with siblings.

Additional Comments:

- The Hemochromatosis Association has suggested that improper creation and distribution of red blood cells and hemoglobin in the body, which in turn produces iron overload or various forms of anemia, is a disease tendency affecting one out of every eight or ten people. The ancient Ayurveda would suggest the same thing. All such conditions are part of the disease of lightness ruled by Mars.
- Surgery is ruled by Mars and, thus, individuals having Mars influencing physical health often turn to surgery as the primary solution for their ailments. If Mars is strong, surgery is often effective; if Mars is weak, surgery may not work.
- The root cause of the disease of lightness lies in high Agni and its tendency to burn the food to a cinder before all the heavy nutrients can be extracted. Such people often eat a large meal soon after they have just finished a prior one. They can't seem to get enough food. At other times they suffer from heartburn. They also suffer from lightheadedness and a feeling that they

are losing their energy faster than they can gain it back. They want more weight and stability in their physiology, but eating doesn't seem to bring it to them. Fortunately, they tend to take a light-hearted attitude towards the whole thing, although, at the same time, in a somewhat driven way. If this sounds paradoxical and hard to understand, imagine a person who keeps striving for something, but in a less than fully engaged manner. This is the behavior of a person with the disease of lightness.

F. T. (Milwaukee, WI)

"I was diagnosed as having 'iron-overload' syndrome by a Western doctor, but the methods for dealing with this problem (blood-letting) were so incomplete that I was getting discouraged. Then Ed explained that I had the disease of lightness, with all of its related symptoms. He instructed me on the various types of therapies which could help me overcome this problem. They are easy to implement."

Case Study

J. came to me complaining of feelings of anger and irritability out of proportion with the situations provoking them. She had been told that she was a Vata-Kapha constitution and had to be careful about taking in substances which had an excessive cold attribute. But cold attribute brings constricted emotions, like fear and melancholy, not hot emotions like anger. She was therefore puzzled over the whole thing. I asked if she ever felt pain under the right ribs (gallbladder) or between the shoulder blades; she indicated yes to both, indicating she had the disease of lightness. The lightness and heat in the gallbladder were causing emotions related to the fire element. With nourishing therapy, she quickly returned to normal and is now as "cool as a cucumber."

The Disease of Heaviness

PULSE: Slow, cold, heavy, large, soft, with low tension, and which can be felt only by pressing quite deeply into the wrist.

URINE: More pale or white in color, turbid, sometimes copious, with sugary taste.

FECES: Must sit for a while before the bowels want to move. Pale in color, sometimes filled with mucus or slimy and watery, whereas in health they are well-formed.

SKIN: Perspires a lot. Skin is cold, white, greasy and plump. Sometimes the person has lipoma formations under the skin.

TONGUE: White coating on the tongue. Tongue may be swollen. Digestion will be slow. The person even eats slowly, wanting to talk after each mouthful. Sweet taste in the mouth. Craving for sweets can lead to diabetes.

VOICE: Slow, deep, soft, depressed, melancholic, but sweet and loyal in disposition.

EYES: Clear and very white, but with tendency to have mucous discharge around the eye. Iridologists will see white lesions in the eye, which indicate the buildup of fat in the tissues.

FACE: Will appear unconcerned and apathetic, although actually the person is quite possessive and earthy. The face may be fat, but even if it isn't, the person will have a heavy expression due to carrying the weight of the world on their shoulders.

ADIPOSE TISSUE: Excess weight in the physiology (obesity), or the feeling of great weight in the psychology (melancholic, depressed, lacks energy). Fat toxins tend to clog the liver. Lipoma appear under the skin. Phlegm can lodge in the ears. There can be abnormal fat growth or tumors, often benign.

CONCEPTION VESSEL: See endocrine system below.

LIVER MERIDIAN: Diabetes, jaundice, hepatitis, mononucleosis, difficulty urinating, vomiting and indigestion, distention in the lower abdomen, and low energy.

ENDOCRINE SYSTEM: Jupiter governs the physiological aspects of fertility: the male sperm and the female ovulatory cycle. Some suggest that the Leydig cells in the male produce the hormones responsible for, or at least related to, male fertility. The female ovulatory cycle is more complex. The important point to note is that the disease of heaviness interferes with fertility.

MISCELLANEOUS: Talking to excess causes a weak feeling in the throat and chest. The person has adhesive mucus, difficult to detach and bring up. There can be twitching in the muscles of the forearm and hand or

Typewriters' paralysis. Respiration can be short and oppressive with cough due to excess mucus in the lungs.

Additional Comments:

- Since this disease is centered in the liver (not recognized by modern Ayurveda), there is often a marked debility that goes along with the other systems. These individuals often feel that their problems are psychological since they suffer from melancholy and depression, but their problem is actually a physical one: the disease of heaviness. Getting such a person to do the right therapies for their illness is difficult, since one of the symptoms of their disease is laziness. They can get fevers due to colds, which are nature's way of cleansing the system of fat.

C.C., (Denver, CO)

"I was quite depressed, but the psychologists were doing me no good. Ed explained that my problems were physical, not psychological, and that I had the disease of heaviness. Through what Ed calls 'lightening therapy,' I have recovered my health as well as my sanity."

CASE STUDY

P. One of the board members of the non-profit corporation which promotes my work was dating a woman, and he asked if I could help her. She complained of having no energy, of being constantly depressed and melancholic. She was slightly overweight, but not to any marked extent. I quickly diagnosed her as having the disease of heaviness despite her weight not being abnormally high. She was given lightening therapy and within two weeks began to feel better for the first time in five years.

The Disease of Dryness

PULSE: Tends to be thready, crooked and slippery like a moving snake, feeble, porous, irregular, tortuous, and vanishing.

URINE: Has a dark brown color, is frothy, scanty, with emission drop-by-drop in advanced cases. There may be frequent, ineffectual tenesmus.

FECES: Constipation with dry, hard, lumpy, black stools. There may be impaction of feces causing obstruction of the bowels.

SKIN: Little perspiration, even on exertion. The skin will be quite dry, especially if the individual has a Vata constitution. There may be cracking and roughness of the skin with a numbed sensation in the extremities. Females may be hypersensitive in the reproductive organs.

TONGUE: Dry, furrowed and red on margin. Finds it difficult to put out tongue and it may tremble if he can do so. Tongue may have slightly bluish or black color or furring.

VOICE: Fearful, depressed, apathetic, with slow or distorted perception. Memory will be impaired, particularly in old age (Alzheimer's Disease).

EYES: Lack moisture and are dull in appearance. The pupils are contracted.

FACE: Looks fearful or depressed. The person has a slightly ashen look with sunken cheeks. There may be tremor in the naso-labial muscles.

MUSCLE TISSUE: The muscles tend to become too contracted and tense. There will be incoordination between the right and left sides of the body with, in severe cases, paralysis, M.S., Parkinson's disease, and hypertension due to sclerotic conditions in the arteries. This disease also causes generalized sclerotic conditions throughout the whole body.

STOMACH MERIDIAN: Tendency to form gas in the stomach with much burping. There can be contraction in the esophagus and stomach with pressure and tightness and even difficulty swallowing solids. Indigestion and pain are common.

SPLEEN MERIDIAN: Gastric pain and abdominal tension, vomiting, constipation, urine retention and weak immunity.

MISCELLANEOUS: Dry hair, tinnitus, excessive colic, loss of sexual power, sclerosed spinal cord, and twitching, cramping, numbness, and coldness in the extremities.

The ancient sages also mentioned that this disease can create problems in the legs, laziness, unforeseen dangers, weakness due to over-exertion and bodily accidents (also related to Mars) through the falling of trees, stones or other heavy objects.

ENDOCRINE SYSTEM: Those parts of the male and female reproductive system which allow us to be sexual without necessarily making us fertile (the second endocrine system related to Jupiter). In the male, this system consists of the prostate. In the female, it consists of the cervix. There may be some other aspect of the female reproductive system which creates the sexual impulse rather than promoting fertility.

Additional Comments:

- This is a classic Vata disease where the symptoms of dryness predominate over coldness (the Moon). The problem always begins in the colon, causing stubborn cases of constipation. The entire physiology and psychology begin to feel contracted and tense. This in turn breeds fear and anxiety, which cause more dryness, creating a vicious cycle.
- There tends to be neuro-muscular problems, and various types and degrees of incoordination.
- Often, the worst symptoms of the disease do not manifest until one is quite elderly (Saturn governs old age), such as in the case of Ronald Reagan, our former President.

B. T.(Fairfield, IA)

"Maharishi Ayurveda is the primary form of Ayurveda used in this town, because Maharishi's university is here. From this system I had always assumed that my health problems were Pitta-related, particularly my severe allergies in the summer. But Ed has convinced me, both intellectually and from my experience in using his suggestions, that my problems stem from the disease of dryness. Oleation therapy has totally relieved my allergies. But I've also seen how hard it is to get the average person to accept this new approach to Ayurveda. People have a lot invested in their paradigms!"

CASE STUDY

L. A woman has a constricted Saturn governing her physical health and thus she suffers from the disease of dryness in its most severe forms. She gets so very depressed and fearful at times, she is virtually incapacitated by her ailments. But she is also a very intelligent woman who is becoming quite optimistic about her health now that she has an effective blueprint to work with, and sees how her mental health is related to her physical health. It is fair to say that her health has improved at least fifty percent in just the few short weeks she has been working with this new health paradigm.

The Disease of Oiliness

PULSE: Heavy, fleshy, soft, sluggish, and slightly slippery. The deep pulses (solid organs) can only be felt with unusually deep pressure, as with the disease of heaviness.

URINE: Sour in taste with an oily consistency. There may also be excess urination.

STOOL: Tendency to loose, oily stool, but there can be constipation when the pancreas is not functioning normally and the person suffers from low or high blood sugar.

SKIN: Acne, psoriasis, itching, profuse sweating, with the skin sometimes acquiring a bluish, marbled condition.

TONGUE: Strong metallic or slimy taste with much saliva. There may be stammering speech with a constant protrusion and contraction of the tongue.

VOICE: Person tends to express fixed ideas and moroseness, and often uses words not intended. There is fear and a sense of emptiness.

EYES: There may be a fixed, staring, glistening look. The eyes may be turned upwards or they may be crossed. The eyes can ache and, in severe cases, become sunken. There may be blurred vision.

FACE: There can be blueness in the lips and face with contracted jaws.

REPRODUCTIVE TISSUE: This disease affects the entire reproductive system in the male and female: prostate and testes in the male and the uterus, ovaries and vagina in the female.

Note: The Moon and the disease of coldness have a primary influence on the uterus and menstruation; Venus' influence is secondary.

BLADDER MERIDIAN: This is a meridian with sixty-seven points on it, so the symptoms are many and varied, but it is particularly useful for abnormal seminal emissions, bladder infections, urine retention, impotence, low back pain, diarrhea, constipation, pain and distention in the abdomen, and mental confusion and disorders.

KIDNEY MERIDIAN: Urine retention, impotence, irregular menstruation, uterine prolapse, diarrhea, constipation, asthma, nausea and vomiting, generalized weakness, and mental derangement.

THE ENDOCRINE SYSTEM: Various types of thyroid imbalances can exist.

MISCELLANEOUS: Spasmodic afflictions, cramps, convulsions, with chronic nausea especially after oily food. There can be epilepsy, meningitis, and chronic spasms in the toes and fingers.

The ancient sages suggested that Venus relates to mental illnesses (physically based, pancreatic and thyroid imbalances), diabetes, leucoderma, sexual and urinary problems, and tiredness and exhaustion.

Additional Comments:

- The disease of oiliness tends to create a thickening of oily substances, which then are deposited in the joints, causing various forms of arthritis. Osteoarthritis is due to wear and tear or poor bone structure, and is not related to the Venusian form of arthritis more commonly known as rheumatoid arthritis.
- Oily, loose stool is one of the first signs of this disease, but it is not an infallible symptom. The same can be said for blood-sugar abnormalities which, in turn, are often related to mental derangement.
- There will be a tendency to thyroid imbalance.

Anonymous (Fairfield, IA)

"I am a Western M.D., trained in Maharishi Ayurveda. I have found this system to be somewhat ineffective in many cases, and did not understand why until I began to consult with Ed about a number of troubling cases. I can think of one particularly striking example when a women with serious ovarian problems was felt to have a Vata disorder and was being given a classic Vata pacifying program. She only got worse from such a regimen. Ed explained that she had the disease of oiliness and recommended drying therapy; she quickly recovered.

I have found that I am able to use this system of knowledge which Ed calls the "Ancient Ayurveda" quite effectively with my clients. It has given me a whole new paradigm to work with, but I am not ready to go public with my discoveries since many of the people in this community might be prejudiced against me for speaking out against their guru's model of Ayurveda."

The Mixed Type of Disease

Note: These symptoms will relate to Mercury uninfluenced by any other planet and, therefore, exhibiting only the qualities of a classical Mercury disease tendency. This means looking at the tissue, meridians and endocrine system related to Mercury. Mercury, when unrelated to any other planet, shows the classic symptoms of Vata derangement.

PULSE: Fast, slippery like a snake, feeble, cold, vanishing, irregular and having other Vata characteristics.

URINE: Dark brown color and frothy. The urine may taste slightly bitter and astringent.

FECES: Dry and hard with darkened, gray or black color. The patient tends to be constipated. Person has a never-get-done feeling, and there can be chilliness with evacuation of stool.

SKIN: Dry, rough, cracked and numb. The color turns dark and the skin feels cold. In severe cases (deficiency) there may be profuse sweating. Mercury governs many kinds of skin problems that stem from dryness and coldness, such as dry eczema.

TONGUE: Dry and furrowed with gray or black furring. Tongue may tremble. There may be spongy, receding gums.

VOICE: Dry, rough and hoarse with sore vocal chords. Speech difficult on account of trembling tongue. Voice is strained and weak (undernourished through Rasa Dhatu).

EYES: Lack moisture and do not shine. Contracted pupils. Lids may also be red thick or swollen in advanced cases.

FACE: Pale, earthy, dirty-looking. There can also be fear, anxiety and apprehension.

LYMPH TISSUE: All types of lymph derangement, including lymphatic cancer, when Mercury is very weak or the person fails to drain the lymph glands through normal exercise.

LARGE INTESTINE MERIDIAN: Constipation, headache, sore throat, aching of shoulders, arms and hands, cough, asthma, and scrofula (swelling of lymph glands, especially in neck).

LUNG MERIDIAN: Cough, tonsillitis, asthma, spasmodic pain in elbow and arm, and generalized pain in the chest.

ENDOCRINE SYSTEM: All disorders of the pituitary gland and hypothalamus, such as abnormal growth and development in a child.

MISCELLANEOUS: Sensitive to heat and cold (a human thermometer), sinus problems, headaches, tremors, shooting pains throughout body, and whooping cough.

The ancient sages relate Mercury to fever caused by the fury of all the doshas, eye, ear, nose and throat problems, skin diseases and mental aberration, and extremely bad dreams.

Additional Comments:

- Mercury relates to lymph tissue, the most basic tissue, which is associated with our overall nourishment. When this tissue fails to function properly, it is the root cause of many other diseases, because the six tissues which are "downline" from the first tissue (lymph) fail to receive adequate nourishment.
- Since Mercury is most often related to other planets, we seldom see a non-mixed or pure Mercurial disease. More often we see a mixed type of disease in which Mercury takes on the disease type of the planet(s) with which it is associated. But the Mercurial tissues, organ meridians, and endocrine gland are

still affected with that disease tendency, whether it be heat, cold, etc., along with the tissues, organ meridians and endocrine glands related to the other planet(s) associated with Mercury.

- Mercury also relates to the nervous system and how well it functions. Nervousness or hypersensitivity can be a symptom of this disease tendency.

Note: It should be clear, by now, why a true science of the stars is invaluable in diagnosing and treating disease, and why health practitioners are handicapped without this true science. However, I must again say that, in my belief, the present practices of both Western and Vedic astrology are not capable of making the types of determinations I'm talking about in this work.

So what is a practitioner to do? He must just treat the symptoms as they arise and hope to peel the onion of disease layer by layer, trying one thing and then another, until something works. He may also consult the New U for a personalized educational analysis (see Resources).

While disease classifications are indeed quite intricate, this paradigm I offer hopefully brings coherence to an otherwise potentially chaotic field of almost an infinite array of symptoms and modalities of treatment.

G. S. (Lake Geneva, WI)

"When Ed explained that I had a mixed-type disease with opposing disease influences (coldness and heat), it sounded complicated but it also fit my experience. So in my program I pay great attention to the seasons. In the summer I treat heat and in the winter I treat cold. It actually isn't that complicated after all!"

CASE STUDY

R. has Mercury, not related to any other planet, governing his physical health. This means his disease tendencies are restricted to the large intestine and lung meridians ruled by Mercury. He complained of great nervous tension and particularly debilitating pains in the neck. He was given a colon cleansing program as well as herbs to strengthen the nervous system. He is doing much better now, but his recovery is still slow due to his weak vital body, which is not easy to treat.

Note: a weak vital body signifies a poor ability to recover from physical illness.

Other Key Symptoms for All Disease Types

AGGRAVATION AND ALLEVIATION: If administering or applying a particular attribute aggravates or relieves a specific health problem, an additional diagnostic clue is provided. For example, if one's headache is aggravated by cold conditions or applications, we can rule out the disease of heat or the disease of lightness. If cold relieves the condition, then we know that the disease of heat or the disease of lightness is possibly involved. Of course, these examples don't apply to advanced cases of humoural deficiency where, for example, heat could be the deficient condition brought on through excess cold.

SEASONAL: Be alert to this seasonal correlation with disease tendency. If a person's allergies strike mostly in the summer, suspect either the disease of heat or lightness.

SEASON	ATTRIBUTES	AGGRAVATES
Fall	Dryness, Cold, Wind	Vata
Summer	Heat	Pitta
Winter	Cold and Damp	Kapha and Vata
Spring	Warm and Damp	Pitta and Kapha

TIME OF DAY: Pay attention to when your discomforts seem to worsen and you will have a good clue as to which primal disease is the cause.

TIME	DISEASE	MERIDIAN
11 p.m. - 1 a.m.	Lightness	Gall Bladder
1 - 3 a.m.	Heaviness	Liver
3 - 5 a.m.	Mixed-Type	Lung
5 - 7 a.m.	Mixed-Type	Large Intestine
7 - 9 a.m.	Dryness	Stomach
9 - 11 a.m.	Dryness	Spleen
11 a.m. - 1 p.m.	Heat	Heart
1 - 3 p.m.	Heat	Small Intestine
3 - 5 p.m.	Oiliness	Bladder
5 - 7 p.m.	Oiliness	Kidney
7 - 9 p.m.	Coldness	Pericardium
9 - 11 p.m.	Coldness	Triple Warmer or Tri-doshic

MISCELLANEOUS: Any part of the body can be a map of the entire body. Thus, some use the ear (ear acupuncture) for diagnosis and treatment. Others use the eye (iridology), the tongue, navel, or the hands and feet.

An Eighth Disease Category

There is an eighth possibility regarding disease symptoms in this ancient science. When the North and South Nodes of the Moon govern physical health, then the person suffers from "demon diseases" — diseases which are due to past life karma rather than present transgressions or mistakes. Such disease tendencies are very hard to diagnose and treat. The two nodes, called Rahu and Ketu in Sanskrit, are shadowy planets which disguise or hide their influence. Since these type of diseases are primarily psychic and karmic in origin, they are best treated through "Yagya" or sacred ritual.

Like Mercury, these planets take on the energy of planets associated with them, and also indicate mixed symptoms and disease tendencies. But in this case the root of the problem is Rahu and Ketu, not the other planets. Let's say Rahu is associated with the Moon and Ketu with Saturn in a proper astrological analysis. Then, in such a case, one must not only treat the disease of dryness and coldness (Ketu representing the underlying disease tendency and Rahu the more surface one), but one must also honor the Nodes of the Moon, since they are the root cause of the problem.

The complexity of this disease complex is another indication of the need for a true science of the stars. This statement may sound absurd to many modern physicians, who are trained to view the body in materialistic terms, however, it may now be time to challenge the skeptics. The knowledge presented in this book comes from an astrological paradigm, which suggests staying open to the possibility that such a true science does exist and has been the basis for resurrecting the ancient Ayurveda.

A. S. (Phoenix, AZ)

"When Ed suggested that I probably had run from healer to healer trying to figure out what was wrong with me, without success, I began to cry. I had become so frustrated by everyone telling me nothing was wrong, or that I was making it up. According to Mr. Tarabilda, my disease type stems from past-life influences and, evidently, these influences always tend to be disguised and not easily treated. I think I have a handle on the problem now, even though I'm not totally better. He warned me that long-standing problems like mine take many months of treatment."

CASE STUDY

A. has the karmic disease tendency due to the Nodes of the Moon and, in her case, this tendency manifests as disguised coldness at the deepest level and lightness at the more surface level. In her case, I emphasized 'Yagyas" or sacred rituals for dealing with her health issues, along with programs for dealing with the symptoms of cold and lightness as they arise. She has indicated that the rituals give her immediate relief, but that the effects wear off after a few months and she must do a new ritual.

Treating the Diseases

Ayurveda, whether we are speaking of the ancient or modern practice, is a holistic health science which treats body, mind and spirit as one unit. Because of this, we should expect the therapeutic aspect of Ayurveda to be quite extensive and comprehensive. How can we get a comprehensive grasp of all the possible modalities open to us in a particular treatment situation?

As shown in the chapter on the etiology of disease, there are nine fundamental causes of anything, including disease: earth, water, fire, air, ether, direction, time, mind and soul. Using these categories as a basis for organizing all the different types of therapy, we come up with the divisions as shown in the chart on the following page.

Of all these possible therapies, some are more important than others. Certainly both ancient and modern Ayurveda place great emphasis on dietetics, herbology and Panchakarma. Ancient Ayurveda includes a homeopathic emphasis as well. Modern Ayurveda uses massage therapy and, sometimes, marma-point therapy as part of Panchakarma. Ancient Ayurveda does not rigidly sepa-

CAUSES	ASSOCIATED WITH	THERAPIES
Earth	Smell	Aromatherapy
Water	Taste	Dietetics, natural medicines (herbology and homeothapy)
Fire	Sight	Color and gem therapy
Air	Touch	Hatha yoga, massage, marma-point, acupressure and acupuncture
Ether	Sound	Mantras (primal sound) and music
Direction	13 basic urges	Panchakarma Avoid suppression of expelling urine, feces and flatus, vomiting, belching, sneezing, yawning, eating, drinking, ejaculating, crying, sleeping, and panting after exertion*
Time	Time of digestion, day, season and life	Preventive medicine and rejuvenation therapy (Part Three)
Mind	Thinking	Psychosomatic medicine (Part Three)
Soul	Consciousness	Reserved for Part three

* Note: This section falls under preventive medicine in Part Three of this book. When the Vayus are obstructed, Pitta and Kapha also become stagnant and toxic. Thus, Panchakarma is seen as a vital purificatory procedure to help open all the channels and restore the flow of each of the five Vatas.

rate marma-point therapy from Chinese Acupuncture and Acupressure therapy (see *The Lost Secrets of Ayurvedic Acupuncture* by Dr. Frank Ros for an overview of this issue) and uses both systems either as part of or separately from Panchakarma therapy.

There are a growing number of health products which seek to balance or treat the meridian systems. One company, Acu-Zyme™, combines enzymes, vitamins and herbs in various combinations for each meridian. There are also some Chinese herb formulas tailored to particular meridians.

The ancient Ayurveda uses Hatha Yoga to treat the seven major disease types in quite unusual and unique ways, which will be set forth in this section.

Color, gem, sound and aromatherapy are not commonly used in modern Ayurveda, but recently some books have described these practices. This book will give a few examples of how to use these less commonly applied therapies for each disease type, along with resources for further study in each area of therapeutics.

The Disease of Heat

DIETETICS: Avoid all hot, spicy, pungent foods and tastes, especially if their *Vipak* (post-digestive effect) is also pungent. Instead, take foods which are cooling and moistening in their effect. This is achieved through salty-tasting preparations. Sea salt is the preferred choice; avoid table salt in the form of sodium chloride. Bitter and astringent tastes are also cooling, but they, like the Sun, are catabolic in nature and thus not as useful as salty taste. One can also take cooling nourishing foods, like cucumber, asparagus, wheat, barley, sweet potato, coconut, etc. Foods listed as decreasing Pitta are all acceptable, but the more anabolic the effects, the better. Eat more cooling fruits, fresh juices, and salads. Solar types must also take in enough water, even when not thirsty.

For a further discussion of how modern Ayurveda looks at nutrition, read *The Ayurvedic Cookbook* by Amadea Morningstar with Urmila Desai.

HERBOLOGY: Avoid heating herbs and emphasize ones from any tradition which cool and moisten, such as Shatavari, Bala, Hibiscus, Aloe Vera, Gotu Kola and Lotus. Herbs which tonify the heart, like Hawthorn Berries and Motherwort, and circulatory herbs, like Prickly Ash, are also useful. One can use purgative herbs to drain heat from the small intestine, such as Dandelion, Yellow Dock, Cascara Sagrada, and Rhubarb. The carrier (*anupana*) of these herbs should be a salty preparation of some sort. Sugar can also be used.

For a further discussion of how modern Ayurveda uses the science of herbology, read *The Yoga of Herbs: An Ayurvedic Guide to Herbal Medicine*, by Drs. David Frawley and Vasant Lad.

HOMEOPATHY: Homeopathic gold, called Aurum Metallicum, is most useful. Certain other remedies, including cell salts, might also be appropriate as part of an overall homeopathic treatment program. Colloidal silver (not a homeopathic but an actual metallic preparation)* is theoretically useful in treating the disease of heat.

*More research is necessary to determine the appropriateness and efficacy of colloidal metals, such as gold and silver. Traditionally, purified or transmuted metals have been utilized therapeutically in India and elsewhere in the Far East.

Note: As a general rule, all homeopathic preparations should be taken between meals, two to three times a day for one week, in 6x or 6c potency. Stop for a month before repeating the same cycle for one more week. If, after a number of months, one feels the need for more of the remedy, repeat the same cycle(s) with a slightly increased potency of the metal — possibly 9x or 9c. I can only give the roughest of guidelines in how to take such remedies; many homeopaths would have very different ideas about the various modes of treatment.

Unfortunately, there are no books at the present time which go deeply into Ayurvedic homeopathy, but if we understand Ayurvedic herbology and how homeopathy is the opposite of allopathy, we can successfully use homeopathy according to Ayurvedic principles. For example, snakebite produces many Vata and Pitta symptoms; thus, in a homeopathic dosage it will relieve Vata and Pitta. Some snakebites give more Vata-type and others more Pitta-type symptoms. Pick a remedy accordingly, or take an herb like Capsicum, which aggravates Pitta, to homeopathically relieve Pitta.

PANCHAKARMA: Purgation therapy to take heat from the small intestine, liver and gall bladder, followed by other forms of cooling therapy. For a further guide to Panchakarma, read *Ayurveda: Secrets of Healing* by Maya Tiwari and *Ayurveda and Panchakarma* by Dr. Sunil V. Joshi.

HATHA YOGA: There are three poses which can be done to balance each disease tendency. The first is always the tamasic pose, which calms, relaxes and purifies any excess due to a particular disease tendency. The second is always the sattvic pose, which balances the system and keeps one from going to unhealthy extremes of either stimulation (excessive rajas) or relaxation (excessive tamas) in regard to any particular disease tendency. The third is the rajasic pose, which stimulates and strengthens any weakness caused by one of the seven aggravating factors.

For the disease of heat, these would be:

Tamasic pose — Headstand (normalizes pineal gland);

Sattvic pose — Tree;

Rajasic pose — Peacock (horizontal and vertical).

MASSAGE: Choose medicated oils which are cooling in nature. Also use types of massage which nourish and cool the body and help the body retain water.

MARMA-POINT AND ACUPUNCTURE: Focus on the heart and small intestine meridians. Do acu-marma points which drain heat and nourish the heart and small intestine. Also focus on points relating to the pineal gland, such as *Adhipati Marma* (crown chakra).

A fine resource which goes into this subject extensively is *The Lost Secrets of Ayurvedic Acupuncture* by Dr. Frank Ros. The marma-points are described and visually illustrated in *Ayurveda and Aromatherapy: The Essential Guide to Ancient Wisdom and Modern Healing* by Drs. Light and Bryan Miller. This book also gives a detailed elaboration of aromatherapy.

AROMATHERAPY: Use essential oils which cool the system, such as rose, sandalwood and mint.

COLOR AND GEM THERAPY: Pastel, mellow colors such as lavender, sky blue, pale pink and pale yellow.

The opposite of the Sun is the Moon, which is milky white in color, so this color is useful.

The gem associated with the Sun is the ruby. Sometimes red garnet is used as a less expensive substitute.

Note: Some gem therapists won't use ruby or red garnet for the disease of heat because they feel these stones are heating and will magnify the problem. Others feel that gems are unique substances which balance all significations related to the planet in question, including its associated disease.

SOUND THERAPY: Intone the "i" sound, as in the English word "ice." Listen to violin music, which soothes the soul and body.

T. D. (New York, NY):

"I used to be addicted to hot tubs because I felt cold all the time. Now I swim in cold water to improve my circulation and I only do the hot tub ever so briefly. I no longer have such aggravated symptoms relating to heart palpitations."

CASE STUDY

D. was a construction worker with the disease of heat, which was aggravated every time he worked out in the hot sun. When this was explained to him, he could think of no solution other than quitting his job, but by wearing long-sleeved shirts and the right kind of hat with a cooling wet towel underneath it, along with some dietary changes and herbal supplements, he can now work construction without detrimental effects to his health.

The Disease of Coldness

DIETETICS: Avoid too much raw food, or large meals which tax the digestive fire. Avoid salty taste and naturally occurring sodium-rich foods. Instead, favor hot, spicy, pungent foods and taste, such as onion, garlic, radish, oatmeal, fish, and chili peppers. Spice your foods liberally and make sure the food is well cooked. Avoid dairy, a lunar food, in all its forms, including butter and yogurt.

Like salty taste, sour taste is too anabolic and, therefore, although warming to some degree, is not an ideal source of nourishment. Lunar types should only drink water when thirsty. They should often drink hot water, especially if sipped at meals, and never take ice water.

HERBOLOGY: All hot spices are useful: cayenne, cumin, asafetida, black pepper, cloves, garlic, cardamom, etc. Herbs which help maintain balanced menstruation are also useful, such as Don Quai, False Unicorn, Red Raspberry and Squaw Vine.

HOMEOPATHY: Homeopathic silver, called Argentum Metallicum, is useful, as is Nitrate of silver (Argentum Nitricum). Colloidal gold (not a homeopathic but an actual metal preparation) is theoretically useful in treating the disease of coldness.

PANCHAKARMA: Use *Swedana* or fomentation therapy, such as sauna and sweats, and include *Garshana* where rubbing with raw silk gloves creates a heating effect on the body. Warm oil packs over affected areas are helpful.

HATHA YOGA:

Tamasic Pose: Shoulder stand (normalizes the thymus gland).

Sattvic Pose: Lotus or half-lotus. Follow with Yoga mudra where one bends forward at the waist, clasps the hands behind the back, elbows straight, and raises clenched hands and arms towards the ceiling.

Rajasic Pose: Eagle.

MASSAGE: Warming oils like mustard or sesame, or heating medicated oils. Use rajasic or heat-producing massage techniques.

MARMA-POINT AND ACUPUNCTURE: Treat the acu-marma points on the Pericardium meridian (also known as the Circulation/Sex meridian) and Triple Warmer meridian. Pay particular attention to those points which are tender. A blocked Pericardium meridian often results in a pathological functioning of the uterus, as well as impairment of the blood circulation and the male and female circulating hormones. It is important to remember that the Pericardium Meridian affects the entire vascular system — arteries, veins and all vessels dealing with circulation of fluids. Pay close attention to points which help activate, purify or balance thymus functioning.

No one needs enzymes more than people with the disease of coldness and its related symptom, low agni. I always recommend the Triple Warmer and Pericardium

Meridian formulas from the Acu-Zyme company, although other formulas are equally useful. Those with the disease of heat or the disease of lightness should be very cautious in their use of enzymes.

AROMATHERAPY: Use warming essential oils, such as eucalyptus, wintergreen, camphor, clove, allspice and cardamom. These oils can also be used on the tender acu-marma points.

COLOR AND GEM THERAPY: Use bright, vibrant colors such as red, orange, yellow, or bright green.

Pearl or moonstone, the alternate stone for pearl, can be used to honor the Moon and the disease of coldness.

SOUND THERAPY: Use the "au" sound, as in the word "sound" or "cow."

A. J. (Sedona, AZ):

> "I bought into the idea that colloidal silver was good for everyone to take. It was supposed to increase immunity, improve digestion, and be a panacea of sorts, so I was taken aback when Ed suggested it was a poison for someone with the disease of coldness. Then I realized that I had really started feeling bad the moment I took the stuff, but had assumed I was feeling bad because a healthy purification was taking place. Now I avoid this cooling substance like the plague."

Case Study

P. struggles with poor digestion like most people who have the disease of coldness, but she was making the mistake of eating a lot of fruit because she felt she could digest it more easily. Uncooked fruit is very cold, especially when taken by itself, and this was aggravating her problem. She had been advised to do this by a naturopath who was an advocate of the raw food program as the basis for healing all disease. It is good to remember that all health problems do not have one universal solution.

The Disease of Lightness

DIETETICS: Avoid foods which are light in nature, like popcorn, leafy greens, millet, or dehydrated, flaky foods. Bitter taste increases a sense of lightness in the body and head. An exception to this rule is when a person is taking strong, bitter purgatives for just one day. This causes such an excess that the system is actually stimulated to throw off the excess.

One should take reasonable quantities of heavy, nourishing, sweet foods as part of Nourishing therapy. This will challenge and satisfy the excessive digestive fire (*tikshna agni*). Meals will also have to be taken more often. Better to take a more frequent number of smaller nourishing meals than one or two gigantic meals, which may cause the agni to become even more excessive in its nature.

Sweet taste does not mean taking excessive amounts of concentrated and rich desserts. It means taking in naturally sweet and nourishing foods such as sweet potato, nuts, seeds, and meat, fowl or fish if one is not a vegetarian. Often it is unwise for someone suffering from the disease of lightness — or any catabolic disease for that matter —to follow a vegetarian diet for an extensive period of time. Sour and salty taste can also be included in moderation. The foods should not be too dry or too hot either, because these attributes increase a catabolic reaction. Too much oil also stresses the gallbladder and must be avoided; this is why sour taste must be used in moderation.

HERBOLOGY: Use sweet tasting herbs, like Licorice, Bala (Indian Mallow), Marshmallow, Slippery Elm, Fennel, Comfrey, and other herbs which have a primarily sweet taste and post-digestive effect. Sour and salty tasting herbs can also be used in moderation. Note: There aren't many herbs with salty or sour taste. Herbs which reduce heat in the gallbladder (bitter purgatives) are quite useful: Dandelion Root, Yellow Dock Root, Cascara Sagrada Root, Rhubarb Root, etc. Herbs which dissolve stones in the gallbladder, or prevent their formation, such as Gravel Root, can be helpful.

HOMEOPATHY: Homeopathic iron is called Ferrum Metallicum. It is most useful in treating this disease tendency. Other homeopathic forms of Ferrum may also be beneficial.

If they ever develop a transmuted form of tin, it could be useful in the disease of lightness.

PANCHAKARMA: Nourishing therapy must be emphasized, along with Purgation therapy. A physician should determine if Blood-letting, which helps balance the various iron-overload tendencies, is appropriate, since the disease of lightness can also cause other forms of anemia which could be severely aggravated through loss of blood.

HATHA YOGA:

Tamasic pose: Triangle.

Sattvic pose: Fish (normalizes adrenal functioning).

Rajasic pose: Crane.

When exercising, conserve half the available energy, i.e. if you could run two miles before total exhaustion, only run one mile. Exercise should leave one feeling nourished rather than depleted.

MASSAGE: Use a heavy, deep and nourishing touch, such as deep Swedish massage, with medicated oils which have a sweet taste and aroma.

MARMA-POINT AND ACUPUNCTURE: Pay close attention to sore points on both the Gallbladder and Governor Vessel meridians. Drain heat and lightness attributes from the Gallbladder meridian — the last points on the meridian (#44 and 43) are useful for doing this. Pay particular attention to *Koopram Marma* on the back at the top edge of the kidneys in relation to adrenal functioning.

AROMATHERAPY: Jasmine, rose, vanilla, licorice, sandalwood, fennel and honeysuckle, and other essential oils which have this same heavy, cooling, sweet, nourishing smell.

COLOR AND GEM THERAPY: Muted, heavy, cool-based colors, like rich emerald green, royal blue or burgundy.

Red coral is used to honor Mars. Some would use blue-colored gems to offset the disease of lightness.

SOUND THERAPY: Use the sound "o" as in "bone" to bring weight and other anabolic effects to the body.

D. T. (Tucson, AZ):

"I am a marathon runner and couldn't understand why I didn't have the endurance of some of my competitors and why I was getting injured and sick so much. Now I realize that I have the disease of lightness. I can't have the same training schedule as many others who run marathons. Now that I train less, I actually perform better!"

CASE STUDY

L. is a long term meditator who has tried to condition her body to eat only one main meal at lunch and one small meal at night. Her health has been deteriorating as a result of this regimen because she suffers from the disease of lightness. Now she is eating four small meals at different times during the day and feeling much better. She is nourishing herself once again!

The Disease of Heaviness

DIETETICS: Avoid all concentrated sweet-tasting foods and substitute bitter ones. There aren't many bitter tasting foods, so one must rely primarily on herbs for bitter taste. However, some leafy greens are slightly bitter in taste, as are a few exotic grains such as quinoa. Avoid large, heavy meals or foods which are too rich. Leafy greens are better than root vegetables. Light grains like millet, corn and rye are better than the heavier wheat, rice and oatmeal. Not only is sweet taste too heavy, but sour and salty taste are also too anabolic in their effect. Astringent and pungent tastes, the two other catabolic tastes, can be used to alleviate heaviness.

How we take our food can affect its assimilation. If we sit over a meal for a long time, eating it very slowly, it tends to create excessive absorption and eventual heaviness.

Fasting is an essential part of lightening therapy, but it usually must be conducted under controlled circumstances because someone with the disease of heaviness often does not feel the initiative or energy to do something "difficult" like fasting. They are also prone to self-indulgence (over-nourishment) and don't like to discipline or deprive themselves.

HERBOLOGY: Use all types of bitter herbs, both as purgatives and as herbal teas. Swedish bitters is a wonderful European formula which can be taken after meals. Some bitter herbs, which may or may not be purgatives, are Neem, Gokshura, Golden Seal, Elecampane, Gentian, Barberry, Juniper Berry, Guggul, Sandalwood, Senna, Scullcap and Chaparral. Avoid all sweet tasting herbs like licorice unless it is used as a carrier in very small amounts.

Note: It is not advised to take any herb or herb formula for more than two weeks without stopping for an equivalent amount of time. Otherwise the body acclimates to the herb(s) and nullifies the effect.

HOMEOPATHY: Homeopathic tin is called "Stannum" in the homeopathic literature. It treats the disease of heaviness. If a transmuted form of iron is ever developed, it might be useful for the disease of heaviness.

PANCHAKARMA: Lightening therapy in all its forms is the therapy of choice. This can include fasting, vigorous exercise, sauna, sun and wind exposure, and purgation therapy (dissolves fatty deposits and relieves liver stagnation).

HATHA YOGA:

Tamasic pose: Spinal twist.

Sattvic pose: Turtle (balances the hormones related to fertility).

Rajasic pose: Cow.

Exercise can be performed until one feels somewhat tired, rather than feeling nourished at the end of exercise as for those with the disease of lightness. If one is obese, then use caution in exercise in order to avoid stroke or heart attack.

MASSAGE: Light alternating with deep, pointed, sharp, heating types of massage should be used rather than more nourishing massage techniques. Dry massage may be in order. The massage need not be enjoyable; let it even be a little painful or uncomfortable. There is an old Ayurvedic adage: "Treat Kapha like an elephant." You can't treat an elephant like a delicate bird or it won't even notice what you are trying to get it to do!

MARMA-POINT AND ACUPUNCTURE: Focus on the Liver and Conception Vessel meridians and any points which are tender or "hot-spots." Remember that vigorous exercise is also very important for good liver functioning as well as weight control. It is not enough just to treat points on the body.

AROMATHERAPY: Use light, sharp, warming essential oils, like Ajwan, clove, camphor, turmeric, sage, and pine.

COLOR THERAPY AND GEMS: Light, pure, clear colors, such as pale yellow, pale pink, lavender and mint green.

Yellow Sapphire or Golden Topaz is the gem for honoring Jupiter. Some would use an opposite color for physical health purposes, such as red coral.

SOUND THERAPY: Use the "a" sound as in "aim" or "blame."

C. K. (Ottomwa, IA):

"I have to eat out a lot due to my work schedule and I always tend to overeat. Ed convinced me to start taking Swedish Bitters after meals to help offset my disease of heaviness. I hate the stuff, but what a difference it makes!"

CASE STUDY

J. is a therapist in Chicago who tends to suffer from depression and fatigue. It obviously interferes with her work. I suggested she treat this disease of heaviness with lightening therapy and especially bitter tasting substances. I have also recommended the trampoline for her workouts. This form of exercise is excellent for individuals suffering from the disease of heaviness. After some initial lethargy and resistance to what I proposed, she is now doing this program and seeing beneficial results.

The Disease of Dryness

DIETETICS: Astringent tasting foods and herbs aggravate the disease of dryness, as do foods which are dry in their nature like popcorn, dry crackers, legumes, and rough leafy greens. Sour taste increases oleation in the body: yogurt, buttermilk, pickles, vinegar, sour fruits, sauerkraut, etc. Lemon and lime are sour and astringent in taste and therefore are mixed in their effects.

Eating while nervous and tense tends to increase dryness in the body regardless of the food taken. We cannot ignore psychological states when discussing dietetics!

As part of oleation therapy, introduce liberal amounts of oil into the preparation of food. In general, sauteing food is better than frying it. One can even take in a tablespoon of oil (sesame, almond, or any other favorite oil) on an empty stomach in the morning. It is suggested that the oil be held in the mouth for a minute or two to mix with the saliva before swallowing it. Then don't eat for at least two to three hours afterwards.

Those suffering from the disease of dryness tend to need mineral and hydrocloric acid supplementation to help improve digestion and immune response.

When the Spleen meridian is out of balance, the person fails to have a normal sense of taste (tongue dryness). Sour taste creates oil and moisture in the system, including the tongue, and can bring back normal taste.

HERBOLOGY: Avoid astringent and favor sour-tasting herbs, like Amla, Sheep Sorrel, Hawthorne Berry, Raspberry (also astringent) and Blueberry (also astringent) with apple cider vinegar as a carrier. Researchers haven't identified many herbs which have a sour taste and this could be a valuable area to explore.

HOMEOPATHY: Homeopathic lead is called "Plumbum Metallicum." This metal, when used in homeopathic doses, relieves the symptoms of the disease of dryness.

If transmuted copper preparations are ever developed, they might be useful in the disease of dryness.

PANCHAKARMA: Oleation therapy is the key for a person suffering from the disease of dryness. *Abhyanga* is a therapy in which warm oil is rubbed all over and massaged into the body for ten to twenty minutes upon first arising. After completing this process, shower or bathe so the oil which has not been absorbed doesn't clog the pores of the skin. Oil can also be taken in the process known as "Oil-Retention Enema" (*Basti*). In this process, the person inserts an ounce or two of oil (raw sesame) into the rectum and it is retained overnight. One can also put oil in the ears, nose, throat (gargle oil), mouth and on the head, body, hands and feet to help bring oleation to the whole system.

If there is stubborn constipation, a combination of laxatives, purgation and oil-retention enemas can relieve this problem.

HATHA YOGA:

Tamasic pose: Corpse.

Sattvic pose: Cock.

Rajasic pose: Bow.

Avoid excessive dry sauna, sun and wind, all of which are very drying.

MASSAGE: Oil massage is useful, as described above.

MARMA-POINT AND ACUPUNCTURE: Pay particular attention to the Spleen and Stomach meridians for sore points and overall flow of energy. Stomach #36 should always be checked for proper functioning.

Note: Individual or combined points can be needled or pressed deeply as in acupuncture and acupressure; two points can be held lightly, as in polarity therapy; points can be massaged with herbal oils and/or essential oils; suction or moxibustion can be applied to any point; or the entire meridian(s) and its flow can be focused upon.

I often recommend the Acu-zyme products for balancing the Spleen and Stomach Meridians.

AROMATHERAPY: Use oily, warm and heavy scents, like musk, orange, anise, fennel, garlic and onion, and vanilla.

COLOR AND GEM THERAPY: Warm, heavy, moist colors like sea green, teal, or misty blue.

Blue sapphire is used to honor the planet Saturn. Some might use Yellow Sapphire or Golden Topaz instead for physical ailments due to dryness.

SOUND THERAPY: Use the "a" sound like in "spa."

S. S. (Milwaukee, WI):

"I always had felt a sense of irritation in my whole system until I started doing oleation therapy in the form of oil retention enemas overnight. Now I feel much more smooth and grounded. Of course, now my diet is also filled with unctuous substances. The program seems so simple and yet is so profound in its benefits."

CASE STUDY

M. is a Kapha body type who suffers from hardening of the arteries and high blood pressure due to the disease of dryness. He needs to take in more oil in order to lower his blood pressure, but had been resistant to doing so because he had been told that this would aggravate his body-type. It hasn't, and now he controls his blood pressure quite effectively through oleation therapy.

The Disease of Oiliness

DIETETICS: Avoid oily foods (especially fried foods) and sour taste as much as possible. Instead, take foods with astringent taste, like legumes, dry leafy green vegetables, pomegranate juice (also sweet in taste), green or black tea and honey, and dry foods like popcorn, dry crackers, dry toast and dried fruit. There are not that many astringent tasting foods and drinks. Primarily use herb teas and decoctions for drying therapy.

Two eating habits to be avoided are lingering over a meal, which produces an overly anabolic effect in the body, and an overly festive attitude, which can generate an oily property in the body.

HERBOLOGY: Use astringent herbs, like Alfalfa, White Oak Bark, Bistort Root, Willow Bark, Boneset, Plantain, Bayberry, Mullein, Guggul, Sage, Turmeric, Mormon Tea or Ephedra, and Agrimony with honey as a carrier. Honey is sweet in taste but quite astringent as well. Thus, even though a person who has Venus governing physical health has a tendency to low and high blood sugar, honey may be safely used for the disease of oiliness. [Note: If blood sugar problems are related to the disease of heaviness, honey may not be appropriate.]

HOMEOPATHY: Homeopathic copper is called "Cuprum Metallicum." It is useful in treating the disease of oiliness.

The metal which relates to Saturn is homeopathic lead. Whether this could be used as a colloidal or transmuted preparation (not a homeopathic) for the disease of oiliness, without creating some form of lead poisoning, would have to be researched.

PANCHAKARMA: Drying therapy is in order, such as *Uttvartna* massage. In this therapy, chickpea flour paste is applied and allowed to dry thoroughly before it is rubbed off vigorously. Dry sauna, dry clay or mud baths are helpful, as are Sunbathing and exposure to high, dry desert wind.

Note: Many oleation practices given as part of Panchakarma by some groups, such as Abhyanga — the intake of ghee to loosen the toxins — and oil basti are contra-indicated and imbalancing to someone with the disease of oiliness. The detrimental effects of using these practices with people who have the disease of oiliness have been documented time and time again.

HATHA YOGA:

Tamasic pose: Plow.

Sattvic pose: Scorpion.

Rajasic pose: Lion.

MASSAGE: See Uttvartna massage under Panchakarma.

MARMA-POINT THERAPY: Treat tender points on the Bladder and Kidney meridians. Put mud, clay, or dry heat applications on any of these points for deeper more long lasting effects.

AROMATHERAPY: Use arid, slightly course, desert-like scents, such as sage, cedar, pine and nutmeg.

COLOR AND GEM THERAPY: Desert colors, like crimson or burnt orange, golden-brown, khaki or olive.

Diamond is the gem used to honor Venus. White sapphire or zircon are sometimes used as less expensive substitutes. Some would use blue sapphire, or other dark, non-variegated colored gems for physical health problems.

SOUND THERAPY: Use the sound "u" as in "boot" or "flute."

A. F. (Duluth, MS):

"My aching joints have never felt so good since I started drying therapy, which basically consists of cleaning up my diet, taking a dry sauna, and drinking an astringent herb formula two weeks out of each month. Why doesn't modern medicine understand these things?"

CASE STUDY

C. was partially bedridden with a severe case of malabsorption and malnutrition. He had chronic diarrhea, which often accompanies the disease of oiliness. Drying therapy took care of his problem immediately with no side-effects.

The Mixed-Type of Disease

If a patient or client does not show the classic symptoms of one of the six major disease tendencies, then suspect the mixed-type of disease ruled by Mercury. How many disease tendencies are involved? How do we judge which is dominant? Look at the predominant symptoms and treat those symptoms. If other symptoms arise, then treat the new symptoms — a process similar to peeling an onion, one layer at a time.

When many of the symptoms relate to the Large Intestine and/or Lung meridians, then suspect this mixed-type of disease. Try to determine whether the disease of heat, cold, dryness, oiliness, heaviness or lightness is predominant in influencing Mercury and treat accordingly. Obviously, such cases are more complicated because we are dealing with at least four meridians (two for Mercury and two for the planet with which Mercury is mixed) and possibly more.

There could even be rare cases where opposite disease tendencies both relate to Mercury at the same time. Without the ability to use a true science of the stars effectively, such cases will always be puzzling to the practitioner. Fortunately, they are quite rare, and individualized consultations are available thru the New U (see Resources).

K. C. (Phoenix, AZ):

"I used to think I was a little crazy, because my health complaints never fit any classic paradigm, including the system I was most accustomed to — the Chinese acupuncture model. When Ed explained how I belonged to the mixed category, and that my case was quite complex, I felt a little discouraged. But now that I am more effectively dealing with these pieces of the puzzle, I'm more optimistic."

Case Study

P. has both dryness and coldness as part of the mixed-disease paradigm. Since these two attributes are both Vatagenic in nature, his case can be treated effectively in modern Ayurveda through the basic program for treating Vata dosha.

The Eighth Disease Category

These cases are even more complicated than the Mercurial ones because they involve a mixed-type of disease tendency, but from two planets: Rahu (North Node of the Moon) and Ketu (South Node of the Moon). The deeper disease tendency comes from Ketu; the more surface tendency comes from Rahu. In addition, Rahu and Ketu bring complaints where the symptoms are difficult to diagnose and treat, as they are due to past life karmic deeds which have manifested in this life.

When this disease tendency is suspected, one must honor Rahu and Ketu through Yagya or ritual and/or through gems. The gem which is conciliatory to Rahu is Hessonite Garnet. For Ketu, the gem is Chrysoberyl Cat's Eye. Then one must treat the symptoms as they arise, while keeping focused on treating the core problem through appeasement.

For example, let's assume that Rahu mixes with the disease of coldness and Ketu with that of dryness. We could treat both these diseases quite effectively and still not cure the person if we don't placate Rahu and Ketu through appeasement. Ritualistic worship of Rahu and Ketu may be done internally as a meditative process, or it may be experienced through a priest or *pundit,* from any tradition, who knows the art of sacred propitiation. Often, only long-term spiritual seekers are comfortable doing their own ritual, but personally-done ritual may be more powerful and effective than that done by outsiders for money. Nevertheless, these "outsiders" provide a valuable service for neophytes in the field of occult knowledge.

T. T. (Chicago, IL)

> "I never dreamed I would be consulting a Vedic pundit for treating a physical health problem, but surprisingly it worked. Of course, I was given other routines as well, but I now see that the core problem is something which lies deep in my past."

CASE STUDY

J. R. suffered from persistent problems with uncontrollable emotions. He assumed the problem was a psychological one, but after many years of using this approach without results, he began to search the physical arena. I suggested that he was in the eighth disease category and that the Nodes of the Moon were causing a disguised liver disease (disease of heaviness). He explained to me that he too had felt, from time to time, that something was wrong with his liver, but tests had never shown any dysfunction, which is often the case in such a disease paradigm. He needed to treat the liver despite the fact that objective science couldn't confirm the diagnosis. Since doing so, he has felt much better. Of course, doing *yagyas* to the Nodes of the Moon was also part of the treatment.

A *CLASSIC* CASE STUDY

W. came to an Ayurvedic clinic complaining of chronic fatigue and migraine headaches, poor digestion and reproductive problems related particularly to the ovaries. She had been diagnosed by a modern Ayurvedic physician as having a Vata constitution and was told her Vata was too high, which, in turn, was causing her major symptoms. She was given the classic treatment for Vata: warming, nourishing, oily foods and herbs and a routine which calms Vata.

Her symptoms became much worse with this program, but she was told that she was just purifying and that in time she would recover. She didn't. Finally she went to see a Western physician, who consulted with me about her case. I explained that she had the disease of oiliness and had been given a line of treatment which would aggravate her disease tendency. I recommended various forms of drying therapy, which the doctor agreed to try. She immediately improved and now leads a normal healthy life.

Note: This is the same case described earlier by the doctor who chose to remain anonymous.

Western Medicine and the Ancient Ayurveda

Today's scientific research in nutrition categorizes people into various types, a process called "Metabolic Profiling." According to this system, people fall into one of three profiles:

1. Individuals who need more protein and fat in comparison to carbohydrates;
2. Individuals who need more carbohydrates in comparison to protein and fat; and
3. Individuals who are more mixed and need an equal balance between protein and fat on the one side and carbohydrates on the other.

Put in terms of the ancient Ayurveda, the first group of individuals are more catabolic in nature (heat, lightness and dryness), the second are more anabolic in nature (coldness, heaviness and oiliness) and the third group are of mixed-type (Mercury, Rahu and Ketu). It is possible to tell which category any individual would fall into based upon an Art of Multi-Dimensional Living analysis described through the principles established in this book.

It is wonderful when modern science can confirm ancient Vedic science. Metabolic profiling is a first step in that direction. I find the comparisons between the two models quite striking and welcome further independent research into their similarities and differences.

J. G. (San Francisco, CA):

"Ed suggested that I have the disease of lightness and need to take in more protein in comparison to fat and carbohydrates. What an incredible difference this one adaptation has made in my energy levels and general well-being!"

CASE STUDY

D. used to eat large meals and feel heavy and lethargic thereafter. He couldn't understand why he would eat so much and yet not feel satisfied. I suggested that he had a catabolic disease tendency (dryness) and needed to take in more protein. He now tells me that he eats less, feels more full without feeling bloated, and has much higher, more sustained energy levels. But he doesn't make the mistake of recommending this diet to everyone. He knows that it is specific to him and one-third of the rest of the population.

Guidelines for Practitioners

The case studies and testimonials presented throughout this book are an attempt to show, in a dramatic way, that the ancient Ayurveda is an already existing, powerful and viable health-care modality. A practitioner can begin to use this model effectively in conjunction with any other medical system of diagnostics and treatment, or by itself. But a word of caution: some knowledge of modern Ayurveda is necessary before one can begin to use this deeper model. I have tried to give the reader an understanding of the basics of modern Ayurveda in Part One of this book, but further study will obviously be necessary.

GUIDELINE #1: First determine the person's constitutional type according to the principles of modern Ayurveda. Then set the results of this analysis aside for later, when you will match the person's disease-type with his constitutional-type in determining the proper therapeutics.

GUIDELINE #2: Take the client's medical history, paying particular attention to the classic eightfold diagnosis: pulse, urine, feces, skin, eyes, tongue, face, voice plus the dhatu(s), meridian system(s), and endocrine system(s) which seem most out of balance.

Pay particular attention to the time of day and season that the disease tendency seems most aggravated and the client's own opinion, if any, as to the cause of the disease.

GUIDELINE #3: Note in particular which attribute seems most aggravated: hot, cold, lightness, heaviness, dryness, oiliness, or some combination of same. Try to slowly eliminate attributes and disease tendencies one at a time.

GUIDELINE #4: Realize that the practice of any of the ancient systems of medicine requires a high degree of intuition, not just the ancient Ayurveda. For example, many practitioners of modern Ayurveda can't agree on the person's constitutional-type. Thus arises the classic joke among people familiar with Ayurveda: "What's your body-type today?"

Another example is the attempt by a Chinese practitioner to determine whether someone is yin deficient or excess or yang deficient or excess. There often can be spirited disagreement in a particular case. Even modern practitioners of Western medicine must use a high degree of intuition when their lab tests give inconclusive results.

So don't be afraid of a system of medicine which requires the substantial use of intuition. At the same time, make sure you are competent to use such an intuitive system before you offer advice.

GUIDELINE #5: Now offer therapy in all the various ways described in this book (both allopathic and homeopathic) to see whether this line of treatment alleviates the condition. If it doesn't, then look at the manifesting symptoms once again and try related therapies.

The following is a guideline and model for determining the specific disease tendency when a true science of the stars is not available.

A woman complains of indigestion over many months. Sometimes food agrees with her, and sometimes it doesn't. Sometimes she feels energy after eating, and sometimes she doesn't. The problem seems to appear during the summer, but she can't associate a particular time of day when it is worse. Lastly, she lives in the high mountains of Colorado. This is all the information she volunteers.

First you can determine her constitutional-type which is Vata and Pitta in equal amounts—a dual body-type. Put that knowledge aside and continue the analysis.

Through the process of elimination, decide which disease tendency is most likely in her case. Start with Jupiter and the disease of heaviness, by asking the following questions: "Do you gain weight easily? Do you ever have liver pain under the right ribs? How do you metabolize fat? Have you had trouble conceiving children? Do you sometimes feel the weight of the world is on you causing you to feel melancholic and depressed? Do you crave sweet taste? Does sweet taste seem to upset your system? Does your voice sometimes sound heavy, and do you articulate your words too slowly?" The client might say that this does not sound like her at all, although of course she can't be sure. So, you tentatively eliminate this disease-type from consideration.

Since poor digestion is sometimes related to the disease of coldness, address this disease tendency next: "Are you cold a lot?" She indicates that she is, but is bothered by the heat as well. "Do you have menstrual difficulties or irregularities?" She responds in the negative. "Does raw food bother you?" She answers that it does not. "Do you sometimes have a sub-normal body temperature?" Again, no for an answer. You can then eliminate the disease of coldness.

Asking her about the disease of dryness, she shows none of the classic symptoms i.e. habitual constipation, cracked or dry skin, poor neuromuscular coordination, hypertension due to arteriosclerosis, melancholy and depression, etc. You might conclude from this that her variable digestion (agni) is not due to dryness in the stomach, or the disease of dryness.

Next focus on the disease of oiliness: "Do oily foods and substances agree with you?" She isn't sure. "Do you gain weight easily?" "Not particularly", she replies. Note that since she has a constitutional type (Vata-Pitta) which predominates in lightness attribute, you cannot rule out any anabolic disease tendency (heaviness, coldness and oiliness) just because she does not gain weight easily. "Do you have a tendency to arthritis?" She replies in the negative. "Do you have blood sugar sensitivities?" Again no. You can then tentatively rule out this disease tendency.

What now remains are the two Pitta disease tendencies: Mars and the disease of lightness, and the Sun and the disease of heat. Ask her if she ever has trouble with her gall-bladder? She says, "yes." "What about anemia?" "No," she responds. "Lightheadedness?" "Yes." "Poor circulation?" "Yes." She also suggests that fiery emotions like anger and jealousy could be there when her digestion is off. You are now hot on the trail! You still have to decide, however, whether it is the disease of heat or lightness which is the major cause of her problem.

At this time, you can take her pulse. Pitta is high both in the gallbladder and liver, and in the small intestine and heart, but it seems a little higher in the latter two organs. Inquiring if she often has heart palpitations, she says yes. Again, this is not conclusive since the disease of lightness can create this same problem, although not to the same degree. When you ask her if she sometimes has feelings of self-condemnation and worthlessness, she gives a resounding yes! Now, you can be fairly certain that her digestive problems are due to too much heat in the small intestine and heart and that she has the disease of heat. You ask her: "How do you handle hot and spicy food?" She indicates that this seems to cause her trouble. Eureka!

You can offer her cooling therapy (both allopathic and homeopathic) to see whether this line of treatment alleviates her condition. If it doesn't, you might look at the disease of lightness once again and try that therapy. If that treatment is less than fully satisfactory, you might look at the mixed or karmic disease paradigm and treat the symptoms as they arise.

The above scenario is actually a case taken from my files. The cooling therapy worked quite well and the woman is now symptom free.

PART THREE

The Search for Maximum Health and Longevity

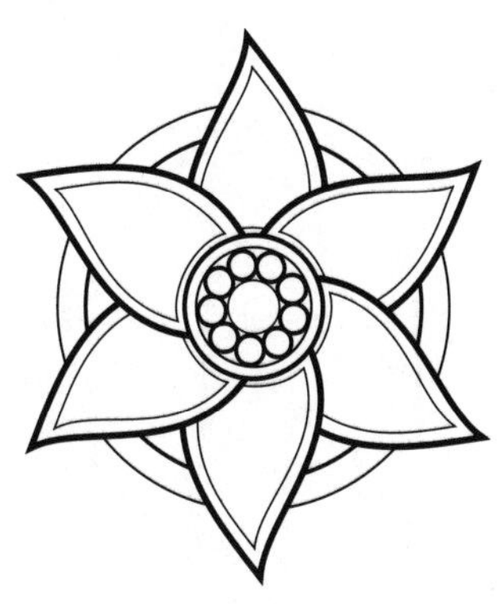

Holistic Living and Its Eight Dimensions

There are myths in every culture which embody the search for physical immortality. The word "Ayurveda" is a combination of two words: *Ayu* means long life and health and *Veda* means knowledge. Ayurveda is the science of how to create a long and healthy life.

We might assume that longevity is determined by mostly physical factors, such as how we nourish our body and how we protect it from pathogens, but research on aging suggests that other factors are far more important in determining who lives the longest — our happiness in career, relationships, and our capacity to sustain a meaningful life purpose.

The Art Of Multi-Dimensional Living would suggest that there are eight fundamental fields of living and that disruption in any of the eight adversely affects longevity. These eight fields are: 1) Spiritual life; 2) Wealth (primal desire nature); 3) Career; 4) Dharma (caste nature); 5) Relationships; 6) Creative Play; 7) Mental Health; and 8) Physical Health. The eight fields of living are not of equal weight or importance. The spiritual life subsumes the other seven fields of living under its primal direction. It gives a person an inner-life purpose.

The field of wealth, along with the other fields, gives an outer-life purpose. When our sense of life purpose (inner or outer) is weakened, then longevity is adversely affected. If we identify ourselves with our career, and it deteriorates, then we often suffer a decline in longevity. If our life is identified with family, and that aspect deteriorates, our longevity suffers as well.

Holistic living is the art of engaging in each field in a balanced and integrated way. This means not becoming identified with any field of living through undue attachment and possessiveness regarding any particular physical or mental object. Non-identification can only be accomplished when the spiritual nature is strong and serves as the focal point for each of the other fields of living. Imagine a wheel: the seven spokes are the seven fields other than the spiritual and the hub is the spiritual. When the hub is centered, the spokes rotate well and the wheel moves forward smoothly and easily. When the hub is not centered, the person gets lost (identified) in one of the seven fields to the detriment of holistic living.

We do not have to be spiritually-minded in order to have longevity. Being driven by an external life purpose may sometimes help longevity because it gives a positive sense of purpose and self-esteem. But more often than not, if we do not have a strong spiritual nature, we will not operate out of our center and will eventually lose perspective. We will begin making mistakes in life and adding to our stress, causing further mistakes. This vicious circle can bring us to ruin, which, in turn, undermines longevity. Thus, a balance of inner and outer life purpose (holistic living) enhances longevity.

We will explore each of the eight fields of living, starting with the field of physical health because, after all, this is a book about Ayurveda and Ayurveda has a primary role to play in our overall life strategy to achieve happy, healthful longevity.

The Field of Physical Health

In the first sections of this book, we have focused primarily on disease and its causes, symptoms and treatment. Properly understood, Ayurveda is just as much a science of health and longevity.

There are three major processes in the universe: the creative (rajas), the preservative (sattva) and the destructive (tamas). These processes define three major approaches to health and longevity:

1. Creating health — through the science of *Rasayana*, which includes various procedures for bringing the fullness of health to the physiology;
2. Preserving health — through various preventive modalities; and
3. Destroying disease — once it arises.

The beginning sections of this book were devoted primarily to the tamasic procedures for gaining health. This last part will focus primarily on the rajasic and sattvic procedures.

Rasayana (Rejuvenation Therapy)

Rejuvenation therapy is one of the eight specialized branches of both the ancient and modern Ayurveda. According to *Charaka Samhita*, which explores this subject extensively, this branch aims at bringing about a number of specific effects:

1. Preventing aging and imparting longevity. This is deemed valuable for its own sake, and also to give the maximum opportunity for spiritual advancement.
2. Promoting immunity. This aim is becoming particularly important because of the depletion of the earth's ozone layer and the build-up of toxic chemicals and pollutants.
3. Improving the mental faculties so one can discriminate clearly and thereby promote holistic health and living.
4. Adding to the vitality and luster of the whole body. This can be particularly important for actors and actresses, models, and other people in the limelight.

In ancient times, most medicines used for rejuvenation were herbal in nature. Today we include not only herbs, but also enzyme extracts, vitamin and mineral extracts, and concentrated food substances like Spirulina or Blue-Green Algae.

Just as Ayurveda focuses on rejuvenation, prevention, and purification for maintaining health and longevity, so Rasayana, itself, has these same three fundamental processes of creation, preservation and destruction:

1. Improving nutrition through formulas which enhance nourishment to all the seven tissues of the body;
2. Improving digestion and metabolism (agni) at all three levels of physiological functioning: gastrointestinal tract, intermediate metabolism, and cellular metabolism; and
3. Improving circulation in the sixteen srotas and/or the fourteen meridians by stimulating, strengthening and cleansing them — another threefold action.

Rejuvenation therapy should be highly individualized, but we live in a world where rejuvenation products are being developed which are supposedly suitable for everyone, no matter what their age, constitution, or lifestyle. In reality, there should be a separate rasayana for each of the seven disease types. The formulas might be similar in some ways, but the herbs and proportions would vary.

Second, there should be variations within each formula for each disease type based on factors such as: 1) constitution; 2) digestive capacity; 3) overall state of tissue health; 4) the state of circulation in the srotas and meridians; 5) the overall vitality; 6) the stage of pathology within a specific disease type; and 7) the overall adaptability within the system.

Third, the age of the patient must be taken into consideration, because each decade of one's life results in the decline or loss of a specific health characteristic:

0 - 10: a certain youthfulness;

10 - 20: the ability to grow quickly;

20 - 30: a certain beauty ("in one's prime");

30 - 40: memory and intelligence;

40 - 50: luster of the skin;

50 - 60: vision;

60 - 70: reproductive capacity;

70 - 80: strength;

80 - 90: thinking;

90 - 100: locomotor functioning.

Thus, if a client is fifty-five years old, he should not only be given a specific rasayana for his specific disease type (altered in accordance with other factors, such as digestive capacity, vitality, etc.), he should also be given a specific rasayana for maintaining or improving his vision. This rasayana could include herbs like Eyebright, Gotu Kola, Jyotismanti and Triphala, taken internally or as part of eyewash formulas.

It is beyond the scope of this book to go into detail regarding the various herbs used in Rasayana. Read *Prokruty: Your Ayurvedic Constitution* by Robert E. Svoboda, and *Perfect Health: The Complete Mind/Body Guide* by Deepak Chopra. Svoboda's chapter on rejuvenation has a very good discussion on the use of metals as Rasayanas.

One of the most famous "universal" Rasayanas is "Chyawanprash." One of the primary ingredients of this formula is Indian Gooseberry, which is very rich in Vitamin C. Another formula receiving some attention these days is "Maharishi Amrit Kalash." This formula was developed by some Ayurvedic physicians who work for Maharishi Mahesh Yogi's world organization. Formulas which claim to promote longevity are a big business and can bring a lot of money into the coffers of the organizations promoting them. They will always have impressive research studies to back up their "wonder-drug" claims, but don't spend a lot of money on such substances too quickly. There are usually less expensive alternatives. For example, Chyawanprash is much less expensive than Maharishi Amrit Kalash and may be just as effective.

Can a rejuvenation formula be used with someone who is in the midst of a disease crisis? It depends on whether the particular Rasayana is compatible with the disease treatment. For example, some Rasayanas use herbs which are then mixed with sugars and made into a very sweet tasting paste. If someone is suffering from the disease of heaviness, this Rasayana isn't efficacious.

The original practitioners of the ancient Ayurveda would have approached Rasayana by creating a separate Rasayana for each disease type. What these more specific Rasayanas consisted of we no longer know, but, I am personally interested in developing reconstituted or new formulas. Other than this one major distinction, the ancient Ayurveda approaches rejuvenation in the same way as modern Ayurveda.

Prevention

The best way to prevent disease is to know the specific disease tendency and the ways to avoid exacerbating it. Applying the knowledge of etiology, we can establish an ideal regimen for maintaining maximum health. At the same time, there are so many suggested parts to the Ayurvedic regimen that only a hermit could comfortably do all of them. A busy householder must pick and choose which regimen he does and when and how he does it. Some aspects of the regimen are quite simple — the kinds of things a mother teaches her children when they are young. Other aspects are more sophisticated. Just remember that the following regimen is an ideal blueprint of ALL the possibilities. It does not require that we do all of them each day.

Ideal Daily Regimen

1. Try to get up before dawn, if you don't feel too tired. Let your body be your guide. Awakening at dawn is natural for animals and primitive people who were fully attuned to the cycles of nature, but not necessarily for today's busy people who have lots of pressure and stress. Dawn is certainly the best time for spiritual attunement, if there is no strain in the physiology from getting up that early.
2. Before going to bed, gently suggest to yourself that you will be alert during the period between sleep and wakefulness. This gap is charged with spiritual energy and focusing on it consciously can create a powerful spiritual upliftment. Once awake, don't dally in the bed. If you fall back asleep when the body doesn't really need that extra sleep, you will feel tired for the rest of the day.
3. Wash the face off with water. Commercial soaps sometimes strip the skin of too many essential oils and acids and should be used carefully or not at all.
4. Drink a glass of water upon arising. This helps the bowels move and cleanses the system of toxins. Then try to evacuate the bowels. If one has

trouble evacuating first thing in the morning, it is often due to staying up or eating too late at night. Excess worry and tension, or certain dietary indiscretions, can also disturb normal elimination.

5. Sprinkle the eyes with purified water or do an herbal eye wash with an eye cup. Dr. Christopher, a famous herbalist, developed a special eyewash formula which many find useful in preventing lost vision or in restoring it. Afterwards, gently rub the eyelids for a few moments.
6. Clean the teeth and stimulate the gums with some dental device such as a tooth-cleaning stick.
7. Use a tongue scraper to clean the tongue. Note: such a device can be purchased in health stores which stock Ayurvedic products. Otherwise, use the long edge of a spoon or a homemade device.
8. Use herbal nasal drops to moisten and clarify the nasal passages. This can be particularly important in dry climates or seasons, or when there is a contagion in the air.
9. Put a few drops of oil in each ear. Mullein oil (squeezed from the mullein flower) is very good for this purpose. Note: some people with a heavy wax buildup in the ears can have problems if they put oil in the ears before removing the wax.
10. Gargle with oil for a minute or so and then swish it in the mouth for a few minutes. This helps the throat, jaw, teeth and gums remain strong and healthy.
11. Pour a small amount of oil onto the head and rub it in. Also rub oil on the feet. If one has the time, rub warm sesame oil over the entire body for ten

to fifteen minutes. Of course, it is equally valuable to have someone do the oil massage for you, but that can get expensive and generally will have to be done later in the day.

12. Follow with a bath.
13. Do some gentle stretching exercises, along with conscious deep breathing, to promote body stability and strength. If one does heavier exercise, bathe after exercising rather than before.
14. Engage in some form of spiritual practice.
15. Try to wear clean clothes every day. Don't wear other people's clothes.
16. The wearing of natural perfumes and pleasing ornaments are highly favored in Ayurveda. They bring a certain refinement of heart and mind highly conducive to health and longevity.
17. Try to wear comfortable footwear.
18. Make sure your clothes, belts, and other accessories are not so tight fitting as to cut off circulation.
19. Ayurveda suggests a special make-up for the eyes called *collyrium,* which also improves the sight. Men in most cultures are unlikely to do this in today's world.
20. Try to have a short period of spiritual practice after work and before one's evening meal to release the stress which has built up during the day's activities.
21. When possible, use the morning for study, the afternoon for more active work, and the evening for celebration.

22. Retire before ten o'clock in the evening if you want to wake up with the rising of the sun.

Ideal Food Regimen

1. A person with a high anabolic tendency should eat only once or twice a day, and never in the evening.
2. A person with a high catabolic tendency should eat when naturally hungry.
3. After finishing a meal, do not eat for at least two to three hours afterwards. Otherwise the natural digestion is disrupted and ill-health can result over time.
4. The quantity of food depends on the power of digestion, the body type, age, and whether one is eating to live or living to eat!
5. Eat according to your disease tendency. For example, if you have the disease of heat, avoid hot spicy foods and drinks.
6. Don't drink an excess amount of water with your meals as it interferes with proper digestion.
7. Either eat in silence or while celebrating with friends, but never eat when in the grip of some negative emotion.
8. Chew food thoroughly. This will not only help digestion, it will also help prevent overeating.
9. Try to avoid dulling (stale) food or food which is overly stimulating.
10. Study various food combinations; learn which ones Ayurveda says to avoid.

11. Review the section on anabolic, catabolic and mixed-disease tendencies and the food recommendations for each type.
12. In today's world, the nutritional properties of food are generally on the decline. You may have to supplement your diet with special foods to offset this deficiency.
13. Water quality is quite poor. Take whatever remedial action is available to you.
14. Air quality is also poor. Take whatever remedial action is available to you.

Note: Don't get lost in the parts and lose perspective of the whole. Food, water and air are the basic ways we nourish ourselves and they are all becoming increasingly compromised in quality. You must be creative enough to offset this triple jeopardy with effective remedial measures in each arena.

Night Regimen

1. Retire before ten in the evening if you want to get up with the rising of the sun.
2. Light, easily digestible food should be taken as early as possible in the evening so that there is a sufficient gap between eating and bed.
3. Try to avoid eating curds at night.
4. Reading at night before bed is a strain on the eyes. Most reading should be conducted in the daylight hours.
5. Avoid sleeping during the day if you are suffering from the disease of heaviness, oiliness, or coldness.

6. Insomnia is caused by Vata and/or Pitta vitiation.
7. To help induce good sleep, rub the feet and head with oil before going to bed. Take warm milk with sugar and ghee. Don't engage in excessive physical or mental activity late at night and listen to soothing sounds before retiring.
8. Learn the various Vedic rules for proper sexual behavior.

SEASONAL REGIMEN

Observe which attributes are predominant during the particular seasons in your locality and act accordingly. For example, if you live in the high mountains of the Southwest, where it gets dry, windy and cold in the Fall, be careful to take substances which alleviate Vata aggravation, particularly if you suffer from the disease of dryness or coldness. If your summers are hot and humid, watch for the aggravation of Pitta dosha, especially if you suffer from the disease of lightness or heat. If your winters are cold and damp, watch for the aggravation of Kapha dosha, especially if you suffer from the disease of heaviness or coldness.

Some countries, like India, are deemed to have six seasons rather than four, with a specific regimen for each season.

Suppression of Natural Urges

Try to establish a regimen and life style which will help ensure that no natural urges are routinely suppressed. For example, try not to establish a business meeting in a way which doesn't allow you to use the bathroom if need be. Try not to get into social situations where you must stifle a yawn or suffer social embarrassment.

The Field of Mental Health and Stress Management

The vital body, subtler than the physical body, coordinates the flow of energy through the physiology so that we feel comfortable. This body also has an effect on our ability to recover quickly and easily from physical illness. During a consultation with a woman who had a very weak planet governing her physical health (Mercury) and a very strong planet governing her mental health and vital body (Jupiter), I warned her about the danger of lymph problems, including cancer. It turned out she had earlier been told by doctors that she had lymph cancer (ruled by Mercury) and would only live a few weeks. She resigned herself to this fact and prepared for death. After three weeks, she was not only alive, but she showed no signs of illness. Her strong vital body was responsible for her miraculous recovery.

When our energy body comes under stress and tension, either through the physical body or through psychological or environmental factors, then we suffer from the stress syndrome: chronic fatigue, tension, negative emotions, insomnia, etc. Stress can come from physical imbalances and Ayurveda exists to take care of that end of the spectrum. Stress can also come from psychological factors and environmental factors. In fact, many emotional problems are due to environmental factors, such as the neuroses suffered by animals who are caged in zoos with no proper space for meaningful activity and interaction.

The ancient Vedic science dealt with stress primarily through the science of geomancy. This is called *Sthapatya Veda* in India and *Feng Shui* in China. Geomancy is the science of how to order the environment around you to maintain a harmonious flow of energy. Some of the main considerations in geomancy are:

1. How to select a site for building;
2. How to locate the home in relationship to the site and the rising and setting sun;
3. The proper location and use for each room in the house;
4. The proper placement of furniture; and
5. How to use certain objects to maximize the harmonious flow of energy within the house — heavy objects, bells, fountains, colored objects, mirrors, fans, etc.

The home is divided into eight sections, based on the eight directions: North, Northeast, East, Southeast, South, Southwest, West and Northwest. Each direction is best for a certain type of activity. For example, East is often the best place to put the main entrance to the house.

When a house is effectively planned according to the rules of geomancy, the person lives in a relatively stress-free environment, which is very conducive to mental health. Of course, it is even better when whole subdivisions are planned in this way, or towns and countries. There is evidence that in ancient days this was often the case. Whether we can restore this type of thinking to our existing cultures remains to be seen. Overcrowded living conditions such as we find in many of today's cities have a detrimental effect on mental health, but, for some reason, we fail to take this lesson to heart in planning our cities' growth and development.

One doesn't need to know all the rules of geomancy to build or furnish a home with good energy flows. Simply let good taste and artistic sensibilities be your guide, or get a geomantic analysis. Every city has a few geomantic practitioners today.

Stress can also be managed effectively through various types of massage or through physical exercise programs such as Hatha Yoga, Tai Chi or Western aerobics.

The Two Aspects of Mental Health

Stress-management is one aspect of mental health, the other is emotional health. I believe it was Mother Teresa who suggested that India had many people who were economically poor, but the West had many people who were emotionally lonely and isolated. Western culture has had a fragmenting effect on its people. Even our celebrations are, more often than not, the passive observation of activities like sports or music. We must once again find meaningful ways to bring people together to celebrate the joys of community.

Aristotle said that humans were, by nature, social animals, but that aspect of our nature has been increasingly threatened by technological advances which have no relationship to family and community living, and which can even threaten it. Witness, for example, the effect of television on family and community life.

Loneliness and depression are bound to have an enormous impact on longevity, regardless of whether or not the person eats well and exercises regularly. Usually, people who are lonely or depressed are less likely to get out and exercise. Everything is interdependent. When we are "down" emotionally, we often don't feel like exercising; we are more likely to turn to junk food to appease that empty feeling inside.

The best way of dealing with negative emotions, which are most damaging to our longevity, is through our spiritual nature. If we can maximize our spiritual potential, then emotional health follows automatically. Negative emotions are undue attachments to some aspect of our life, and true spiritual training nips these attachments in the bud.

The Field of Spiritual Life

Of all eight fields of living, this field is by far the most important — the king amidst the cabinet. To a materialist, any so-called mental or spiritual process is merely an epi-phenomenon of matter. He believes matter to be the cause of all involution and evolution of mental processes, rather than the other way around. On the other hand, an ancient sage would say that spirit wills itself into mind and matter for the express purpose of allowing mind and matter gradually to take more and more part in spirit. Interestingly enough, scientific materialism led to the discovery of quantum physics, which is now undermining the very ground which materialism has stood on so comfortably for all these years.

Spiritual life itself has been undermined not only by materialists, but also by those who try to promote one form of spirituality for everyone. The ancient Vedic teachers were very wise — they recognized that people have different strengths of personality. This, in turn, lead to different approaches in defining and finding the spiritual goal of life. But today's religions are quite exclusive, often condemning approaches other than their own. The same holds true for many spiritual teachers and their teachings: they try to give one generic approach — the "best" way. In theory they may honor all paths, especially if they are from the East, but, in practice, they violate the multi-dimensionality of the Vedic approach.

According to The Art Of Multi-Dimensional Living, there are eight archetypally distinct approaches to finding God or enlightenment, based upon the eight aspects of personality. The tradition which has best preserved some knowledge of these paths is the ancient Vedic path of yoga. In mentioning these various "Yogas," I am not suggesting that this tradition has a monopoly on this knowledge. The core of each of the eight paths can be found in every religious and spiritual tradition. I merely use these Vedic terms because they are the easiest to access in the spiritual literature.

The Eight Approaches to Spirit

1. THE PHYSICAL BODY: *HATHA YOGA* — the path of physical purification and silence.

2. THE SENSES: *RAJA YOGA* — the path of beauty and art. Transcendental Meditation© is a good example of this path.
3. THE MIND: *KARMA YOGA* — the path of selfless service and giving.
4. THE INTELLECT: *JNANA YOGA* — the path of discrimination through the intellect.
5. THE WILL: *LAYA* OR *KUNDALINI YOGA* — the path of the warrior.
6. THE HEART: *BHAKTI YOGA* — the path of personal devotion.
7. THE INTEGRATING FACTOR: *SURYA YOGA* — Integral Yoga, the path which seeks to combine the yogas into one integral practice.
8. EACH PERSON'S UNIQUENESS: *TANTRA* — the path of the rebel or spiritual outlaw.

Each person is meant to use his or her strength of personality and the Yoga which relates to it as their predominant spiritual approach. They may also decide to study the other Yogas and incorporate some of these practices as well, but not at the expense of their primary path. There are two exceptions to this general rule: 1) if one is a Surya Yogin, then no one path is predominant — all of them are combined into one integral practice; and 2) if one is a Tantric, then one's practices cover the full range of all Yogic techniques, but in a highly unorthodox and experimental way. The Tantric's path may appear to be just the opposite of Yoga because it utilizes desire in a conscious way rather than controlling or sublimating it.

If religious and spiritual teachers fully honored this multi-dimensional approach to spirituality, then all would be well. They frequently don't. Instead these teachers often tend to foist their own approach onto all the disciples, regardless of individual make-up. A teacher of Bhakti Yoga may try to make everyone else a Bhakti practitioner; a teacher of Jnana Yoga may try to make everyone into a Jnana practitioner. To my mind, this is a real perversion of the deeper spiritual knowledge which lies at the core of all ancient traditions. Know your own strength of personality and then find a teacher who can best serve you. This is a key life strategy in this field.

Any strategy which seeks to bring about physical longevity will only be partially effective if it does not address the field of spiritual life. Without a proper spiritual foundation we keep on making mistakes in all the other fields of living, either through commission or omission. This is why Christ said: "Seek ye first the kingdom of God and all else will be added unto you." The Vedic sages said: *Yogastah Kuru Karmani* —"Establish Being (your true spiritual nature), then go out and perform action in the world." This is why we must constantly emphasize the role of spirituality in relation to happy and healthful longevity.

You may say: "I know many healthy people who aren't even slightly spiritual." I can only suggest that your vision may be too shortsighted. For one thing, spiritual people don't always appear spiritual or religious to others. For another, karmic consequences can extend beyond the death of this body into future lifetimes, but we aren't in a position to see how mistakes in one lifetime manifest in another. Not that you have to accept the idea of reincarnation to benefit from anything said in this or other chapters. The great Lord Buddha himself kept quiet when asked about the subject of reincarnation; he was more interested in ending people's suffering in this life than in metaphysical debates about past and future lives. I feel the same way.

What is important is that there is a definite relationship between spiritual life and health and longevity.

The Field of Wealth

The deepest part of our personality, the field of spirituality, is intimately linked to the timeless, spaceless and causeless Reality which is our true nature, but which we deny through identification with various internal and external objects of perception. When we relax and totally accept ourselves, we sink into who we truly are. This happens most easily through our greatest strength of personality, whether it be the senses, heart, will, mind, intellect, body or the integrating factor in the personality.

There is another part of our personality which seeks temporal satisfaction in the realm of space, time and causality. It too can lead us to ultimate fulfillment by gradually showing us, through many varied experiences, that temporal fulfillment is always partial and always leads to new needs and expectations, which, in turn, lead to other partial and transient satisfactions.

According to all the ancient teachers, this chain of activity — where we desire something, seek to fulfill it, and then desire something else again — leads to suffering. The way out of suffering is to recognize the basic falseness of the idea that there is an agent or actor engaging in some activity to achieve some object. To do this successfully, we must know how to use our inner strength of personality to strip away our thinking that there is an actor, action, and object acted upon.

Such a concept is necessary in conducting ourselves in the world of empirical reality. But that world is different from our real nature, where no agent, actor, and object of action exist. It is this nature, which at some point we are destined to realize in the innermost depths of our being, which fulfills us in a permanent way. At least this is the teaching of *Advaita Vedanta*, the highest system of Indian Philosophy. In the meantime, it is our desire nature which keeps pushing us towards ultimate fulfillment through the disappointments of temporal fulfillment. This desire nature can also be called the field of wealth. Whether we consider ourselves wealthy is more a question of whether we can fulfill our basic desires than any objective standard established by others.

The problem is that the small and petty human ego is intimately tied to the desire nature, and this ego is constantly trying to convince us that temporal fulfillment will actually bring permanent happiness! In this sense, the planet governing our desire nature is the planet which indicates how and where our self-delusions are likely to manifest. The desire nature is the great seductress, always promising more than she delivers. However, the desire nature should not be suppressed, because then we will not learn the lessons she brings us. Neither should the desire nature be trusted, because then she is likely to fool us.

For example, a person who has Venus governing the desire nature often assumes that the spiritual practices related to Venus, such as finding a ideal love relationship or practicing Raja Yoga, are the best means for finding God. In reality, it is the planet which governs the inner spiritual nature which actually provides the clues about which activities are most suitable for each person to find God, but the desire nature often tries to usurp this role. Eventually, a person comes to realize this through hard experience, but by then it may be too late in this life. The sages used the ancient science of the stars to help people make these subtle distinctions, but over time, this ancient science has become so distorted and watered down as to mostly lose its efficacy.

The most essential temporal desire related to each planet is:

The Sun: leadership in one's group.

The Moon: nourishment of others.

Mars: power over self, first and foremost, and then over others.

Mercury: effective communication.

Jupiter: meaningful social interaction.

Venus: ideal love relationships.

Saturn: security.

The Nodes of the Moon: individual uniqueness.

This field of living also has a relationship to how well we hold onto what we value as wealth. If the planet governing this field of living is strong, then we hold onto our wealth quite well. If it is weak, then we squander our wealth. Loss of wealth causes great frustration.

It creates an inner friction and insecurity which can be very detrimental to health and longevity. This is why many individuals suffer a rapid physical decline after losing all their money or possessions, especially if they don't have a strong spiritual nature which helps keep these types of events in perspective.

As everyone knows, wealth can be a blessing because the individual who possesses it can buy anything he or she wants. It can also be a curse because each fulfillment is only partial and leads to another pressing desire. The wealthy can acquire anything they need or want and still be most unhappy! Wealthy people often suffer more than the poor because they no longer have the illusion that money will relieve their sense of emptiness.

Thus, it becomes quite important that we learn to be the master of our desires. If we don't rule them, they will certainly rule us. This is best accomplished through our spiritual nature, which teaches us how to control our desire nature, how to distinguish partial from total fulfillment, and how to achieve total fulfillment.

The Field of Dharma

One of the meanings of the Sanskrit word *dharma* is an action which is moral, ethical and evolutionary for our life. Philosophers have taught that morality is relative, subject to differing opinions, but the ancient Vedic sages suggested that an action is moral when its purpose is to selflessly serve and give to others. The sages then suggested that the best way to ensure that our actions serve others is to know and practice our "caste nature" to the best of our ability.

The word "caste" has a negative connotation in the West, because we have seen the abuses of the caste system in India, where one must accept the caste of one's parents regardless of one's own predispositions and inclinations. This perverted form of caste has never been supported by the sages of India. When they speak of the caste system, they are referring to a society whose members understand their various social and individual natures, a society that freely allows each individual to find his or her place within this system.

Such a knowledge can only be preserved in a society that has a true, profound and fully integrated science of the stars. Such a system has not existed in India for a long time — at least as long as the rigid caste system of India has existed, which may be three to four thousand years or longer. The present caste system of India is living proof that the true science of the stars was lost in India a long time ago, because one of the primary purposes of this science was to help individuals know their caste nature.

There are five possible castes:

Brahmin — priest, counselor and scholar;

Kshatriya — warrior and ruler;

Vaishya — merchant, artisan or husbandman;

Sudra — servant; and

Outcast or untouchable.

The real meaning of an "outcast" is someone whose moral duty is to purify society of its outmoded, outdated conventions and institutions by acting as a rebel or outlaw. This type of person is an outsider and thus often feared by those within the system.

Sudras are those who want to remain free of too much duty and responsibility towards society and who, therefore, volunteer their services to one of the other castes for a period of time. This caste is not servile in any way because Sudras need to protect their independence. Sometimes they can be convinced to take on duties they should have refused, and they must learn to serve in a way that does not compromise their freedom. They need large doses of this freedom so that they can enjoy "the good life." A Sudra is comparable to a spiritual hermit, except the Sudra retreats or hides from externally imposed social duty and responsibility rather than the social life itself.

Brahmins primarily relate to the cultural-religious-educational institutions of society by upholding the value of liberty in these arenas. Kshatriyas relate to the legal and political systems, where they uphold the value of equal rights. Vaishyas uphold the value of fraternity in the economic institutions. Thus, with the first three castes, we have the full development of the three great societal values: liberty, equality and fraternity. Sudras serve one of the other three castes and take on the values of whatever caste they are serving. Outcasts are outside the whole caste structure and live on the actual or psychological fringes of society. Gypsies or hobos are a modern day version of the outcast.

Unlike many East Indians, individuals in the West are free to experiment in order to find their caste nature, but this may take most or all of a lifetime. Thus, some sages suggest that the understanding of caste nature, as well as the ability to use it effectively, is almost as hampered in the West as it is in the East. The Art Of Multi-Dimensional Living provides a way for people to know their caste nature and, therefore, know how to meet their duty to society.

When we wake up in the morning with some burning question as to how to best serve society, we are in the field of dharma. Our dharma is not our career nature, but it is the platform upon which we build a career. Our career nature and our dharmic nature should always be harmonized or correlated for maximum effectiveness in life.

For example, those whose career nature is governed by the Sun will have leadership ability. But where that leadership should be exercised is determined by the dharmic nature. Thus, a Kshatriya should take leadership positions in the government or the military, whereas a Vaishya should do so in the field of business and a Brahmin in the field of knowledge. When a person does not feel that they are "pulling their weight" in terms of helping others, it can result in great dissatisfaction or frustration. This, in turn, can effect health and longevity. In fact, according to scientific research, job satisfaction is an extremely important significator for longevity. It is not possible, therefore, to promote health and longevity in a holistic manner without considering a person's relationship to the field of living called dharma.

The Field of Professional Life

When we meet strangers, we often ask, almost immediately, what they do for a living. When life is meaningful, because we feel that we have an important role to play in it, then our resistance to disease is strong. We have good immunity. When we are bored and listless, then our immunity goes down.

Some individuals are so identified with their work that they don't know what to do with themselves upon retirement, especially if they haven't cultivated hobbies. Such a person can suffer loss of self-esteem upon retirement and the negative health consequences of that loss. Self-love is very important for health and longevity. In ancient times, there was a clear understanding that one's last years should be devoted to intense spiritual practice and preparation for the transition to the after-life. It was anticipated as the most precious time in one's life. This attitude and skill in using one's time spiritually is far less common today.

One of the tragedies of the modern materialistic age is the fact that old people often do not have adequate spiritual resources to fall back on when their external duties are finished. There may be more opportunities for recreation today, but this often leaves the participant feeling hollow and empty afterwards. Oftentimes, children and grandchildren live far away and, thus, the important role of being a grandparent is not fully exercised, or comes into play only minimally. "There must be more to life than this!" is a heartfelt cry for a connection to the spiritual.

Men and women who have the types of careers they can continue on a full or part time basis, even in old age, are fortunate indeed. So we should not be surprised when we find that career satisfaction is a leading predictor of longevity. Someone who continues to work in a job which they intensely dislike does not understand just how harmful this can be to their health and should seek career counseling. The most effective form of career counseling used to be astrological in nature, but these days individuals must rely on Western scientific approaches, which are anything but precise and cannot deal effectively with individuals who have weak career natures.

The astrological science I practice is capable of helping people know with precision their career path and its various strengths and weaknesses. Fortunately, none of the knowledge presented in this book depends on accepting anything I say about astrology. Nevertheless, I feel the issue of effective career counseling needs to be given more attention by both the educational institutions training students and the companies and institutions which eventually employ these students.

The Field of Relationships

When we sense a person is suffering in some way, how often we find it is due to some faulty relationship or interaction with a spouse, parent, child, relative, friend or enemy. Poorly functioning relationships drag us down both physically and mentally, whereas good relationships are catalysts for renewed vitality, bringing a sense of peace and harmony to our existence. Good friends should be cherished above all else.

Seminars on improving our interpersonal and love relationships are rampant in the United States. There is a relationship guru on virtually every corner anxious to teach us how to get along better with those around us, and how to receive what we want from relationship. Much of this information is useful, although often taught in an overall context, I suspect, that reinforces the limitations of the ego. The emphasis should be on helping others meet their needs rather than the more egoic preoccupation of having others meet our needs.

There are seven or eight major styles of relating, which correspond to the eight planets, and each person is predominantly geared towards one of these styles. A style is not good or bad; it is just a style. However, it may or may not be compatible with another's particular style. One person may be solar — a charismatic type who relates well in front of crowds. Another person may be more lunar, with a natural ability to be gentle, compassionate and empathetic in relationship. A style ruled by Mars will be very direct, even aggressive at times, whereas a Mercurial style will emphasize the virtues of flexibility, adaptability and playfulness. A Jupiter style will exhibit fair-mindedness and a desire to serve. Saturn's style will be more reserved and terse, whereas the Nodes will exhibit a rebellious streak.

None of these styles are bad, unless the planet governing a style is weak or malefic in nature. The key is to understand and accept who we are in our style of relationship, rather than thinking there is some universal norm for everyone to follow, such as "men are like this and women are like that." There are some basic biological and psychic differences between men and women, but there are also great variations within each gender. The archetypal nature of these variations needs to be more emphasized.

Sometimes a person's health begins to improve immediately when a certain relationship ends. This is tangible proof that, in the quest for happy, healthful longevity, we cannot ignore our interactions in the field of relationships.

The Field of Creative Play

The field of creative play refers to how we recreate and play. The word "recreation" suggests that play is necessary to help us restore and regenerate our psychological faculties and physical energies. If we used our spiritual nature more effectively, we would not need so much time for play; we would not take everything so seriously and get "burned out" pursuing goals in such a driven way. Action would be performed in a spirit of selfless service and giving, and would be engaged in without attachment to the fruit of the action.

However, we live in a materialistic society where people "compete for turf," and, in the process of doing so, get very tired. Thus, a great need for play arises. But tired people have an overall awareness which is also tired or dull, and, consequently, such people often lack creativity. They make mistakes in how they play: they drink too much or play too hard and, as a result, incur more stress through an activity which was supposed to relieve stress! This is madness, but it is a form of madness which is very prevalent in our society. Witness, at one extreme, the fights that often break out after a sporting event, and, at the other extreme, the passive nature of so much of our entertainment, which has the effect of dulling rather than enlivening consciousness.

One reason we must learn the art of play is so we can raise our children well. A good parent can enter the world of children through a proper sense of play. When we are unable to play effectively, then there is no safety-valve for releasing the constant stress to which the body is subjected to and stores in the nervous system during the course of a week, month, or year. This imbalance in the field of creative play can seriously damage our quest for happy, healthful longevity, just as imbalances in any of the other seven fields of living can do so.

Conclusion

The ancient Ayurveda is a profound understanding of not only the body and the physical causes and symptoms of its health or derangement, but also the other causes which extend into our mental, social and spiritual life. No individual is an isolated entity; we exist in a matrix of processes and events which span seven other fields of living. Only a clear grasp of these other fields, and their relationship to physical health, ensures a holistic and successful approach to health and longevity.

The ancients understood this far better than we do today, and we can learn a lot from them in this regard. But we tend to be so caught up in the frenetic activity of the world, and its increasingly fragmented approaches to problems, that we often turn a deaf ear to the wise teachers of ages gone by. This is a mistake, just as it is a mistake to trust these ancient teachers blindly with regard to modern day problems which, in some cases, need modern solutions. We must learn to distinguish these two very different situations and act accordingly. Hopefully, this book is a first step in that direction.

I have tried to show the value of the ancient Ayurveda for modern health problems without denigrating either modern Ayurveda or the great accomplishments of modern medicine, especially in treating traumatic injuries and acute illnesses. At the same time, I feel strongly that not only modern Western medicine, but also the more modern system of Ayurveda, can benefit a great deal from studying the more ancient model of Ayurveda set forth in this book.

To know your primal disease type, and how to manage it, is the most important first step in health-care treatment, whether that treatment is preventive, curative or restorative. To this purpose I dedicate this book.

BIBLIOGRAPHY

Ballentine, Rudolph. *Diet and Nutrition: A Holistic Approach.* Honesdale, Pennsylvania: Himalayan International Institute, 1978.

Charaka Samhita (Text with English Translation by Dr. R.K. Sharma and Bhagwan Dash, Chowkhamba Sanskrit Series Office, Varanasi, India, 1977, distributed by Lotus Light, Twin Lakes, Wisconsin.

Chopra, Deepak. *Perfect Health.* Harmony Books, New York, New York, 1991.

Dash, Bhagwan. *Fundamentals of Ayurvedic Healing.* Bansal and Co., Delhi, India, 1978, Distributed by Lotus Light, Twin Lakes, Wisconsin.

Donden, Yeshi. *Health Through Balance: An Introduction to Tibetan Medicine.* Snow Lion Publications, Ithaca, New York:, 1986.

Frawley, David. *Ayurvedic Healing.* Passage Press, Salt Lake City, Utah:, 1989.

Frawley, David, Vasant Lad. *The Yoga of Herbs.* Lotus Press, Twin Lakes, Wisconsin, 1986.

Heyn, Birgit. *Ayurveda: The Indian Art of Natural Medicine and Life Extension.* Healing Arts Press, Rochester, Vermont, 1990.

Joshi, Sunil V. *Ayurveda and Panchakarma.* Lotus Press, Twin Lakes, Wisconsin, 1997.

Lad,Vasant. *Ayurveda: The Science of Self-Healing.* Lotus Press, Twin Lakes, Wisconsin, 1984.

Miller, Light and Bryan, *Ayurveda and Aromatherapy*. Lotus Press, Twin Lakes, Wisconsin:, 1995.

Morningstar, Amadea. *The Ayurvedic Cookbook*. Lotus Press, 1990. Twin Lakes, Wisconsin, 1990.

Ros, Frank. *The Lost Secrets of Ayurvedic Acupuncture*. Lotus Press, Twin Lakes, Wisconsin:, 1994.

Sachs, Melanie. *Ayurvedic Beauty Care: Ageless Techniques to Invoke Natural Beauty*. Lotus Press, Twin Lakes, Wisconsin:, 1994.

Sharma, Narayan. *Arogya Prakash*. Baidyanath, Calcutta, India: Distributed by Lotus Light, Twin Lakes, Wisconsin.

Sushruta Samhita. (English Translation by K.L. Bhishagratna, Chowkhamba Sanskrit Series Office, Varanasi, India, 1981.

Svoboda, Robert E. *Prakruti: Your Ayurvedic Constitution*, Geocom Limited, 1988. Distributed by Lotus Light, Twin Lakes, Wisconsin.

Svoboda, Robert and Lade, Arnie. *Tao and Dharma: Chinese Medicine and Ayurveda*. Lotus Press, Twin Lakes, Wisconsin, 1995.

Tiwari, Maya. *Ayurveda: Secrets of Healing*. Lotus Press, Twin Lakes, Wisconsin, 1995.

Udupa and Singh, Editors. *Science and Philosophy of Indian Medicine*. Calcutta, India: Baidyanath, 1978. Distributed by Lotus Light, Twin Lakes, Wisconsin.

Thakkur, Chandrasekhar. *Kaya Kalpa*. Ancient Wisdom, Bombay, India, 1980.

Tierra, Michael. *Planetary Herbology*. Lotus Press, Twin Lakes, Wisconsin, 1988.

Young, Arthur M. *The Reflexive Universe: Evolution of Consciousness*. Robert Briggs Associates, San Francisco, California, 1976.

RESOURCES

The New U

The New U is a non-profit, tax-exempt corporation whose prime purpose is to promote "The Art of Multi-Dimensional Living", a new subjective discipline founded by the author, Edward Tarabilda.

For a list of books, tapes and courses offered by The New U, or for a free brochure on The Art of Mullti-Dimensional Living, write to:

The New U
P.O.Box 751
Fairfield, Iowa 52556
(515) 472-3809

Web Site

www.dimensional.com/~risaacs

One can access or order Edward's book entitled *The Spiritual Labyrinth: Alternative Roadmaps To Reality,* through this site.

"The Global Oracle: A Spiritual Blueprint of Life"

This is a book written by Edward Tarabilda and Doug Grimes which creates a contemporary oracle for prediction and guidance in one's daily life choices. For further information or to place an order contact:

Sunstar Press
116 N. Court St.
Fairfield, Iowa 52556
1-800-532-4734

Correspondence Course

The Art of Multi-Dimensional Living, founded by the author Edward Tarabilda, presents a correspondence course in Spiritual Science. It targets those individuals who want to study this subject in a climate which is non-authoritarian, non-hierarchical, non-invasive, yet personal and somewhat informal. There are 224 principles which constitute this science: 112 which set forth archetypal distinctions and differences in life and 112 processes which transcend and unify those differences. An opportunity exists for the course participant to receive personal guidance as to his predominant strength of personality and its precise use as a spiritual tool. Thus, the student receives both theory and practice, knowledge and experience, universal principles and precise personal applications.

The course is best suited to independent spiritual seekers who are no longer satisfied with the traditional guru/disciple, or other authoritarian models for spiritual training and development. For more information, or to order the course, please contact:

The New U
P.O.Box 751
Fairfield, IOWA 52556
515-472-3809

Consultations

Clients or health practitioners who would like to work with Edward one on one for further support in implementing this knowledge are encouraged to schedule a consultation by calling (515) 472-3809, or by writing to:

The New U
P.O.Box 751
Fairfield, Iowa 52556

Seminars in Pulse Diagnosis

Edward offers to Ayurvedic health practitioners an opportunity to study an advanced form of pulse diagnosis particularly suited to the ancient model of Ayurveda presented in this book. This knowledge is difficult to transmit through writing and is best learned in a "hands-on", small-group format. To schedule such a seminar write to:

The New U
P.O.Box 751
Fairfield, IOWA 52556
515-472-3809

Courses Through The Institute for Wholistic Education

Ed was a leading figure in the creation of two Ayurvedic correspondence courses now offered by the Institute. The first level course trains people to be Ayurvedic

Health Educators. Its focus is the modern Ayurveda explored in the first part of this book. The second level course trains people in the use of the ancient Ayurveda set forth in the second part of the book. For further information about these courses, please write to:

Institute for Wholistic Education
33719 116th Street, Box AR
Twin Lakes, Wisconsin 53181
(414) 877-9396

Ayurveda Centers and Programs

American Institute of Vedic Studies

P.O. Box 8357
Santa Fe, NM 87504-8357
(505) 983-9385
(505) 982-5807 (Fax)

The Ayurvedic Institute

11311 Menual N.E.
Albuquerque, NM 87112
(505) 291-9698
(505) 294-7572 (Fax)

California College for Ayurveda

135 Argall Way, Suite B
Nevada City, CA 95959
(916) 265-4300

The Chopra Center for Well Being

7590 Fay Avenue, Suite 403
LaJolla, CA 92037
(619) 551-7788
(619) 551-7811 (Fax)

Rocky Mountain Ayurvedic Health Retreat

P.O. Box 5192
Pagosa Springs, CO 81147
(800) 247-9654
(970) 264-9224

SOMA

P.O. Box 328
Pagosa Springs, CO 81147
(970) 264-6326

Vinayak Ayurveda Center

2509 Virginia, NE
Albuquerque, NM 87110
(505) 296-6522
(505) 298-2932 (Fax)

Ayurvedic Herbal Suppliers

Bazaar of India Imports, Inc.

1810 University Avenue
Berkeley, CA 94703
(800) 261-7662

Internatural

33719 116th Street-AR
Twin Lakes, WI 53181
(800) 643-4221
(Retail mail order supplier of Ayurvedic books and herbal products)

Lotus Brands, Inc.

P.O. Box 325-AR
Twin Lakes, WI 53181
(414) 889-8561
(414) 889-8591 (Fax)

Lotus Light Natural Body Care

P.O. Box 1008-AR
Silver Lake, WI 53170
(414) 889-8501 or (800) 548-3824
(414) 889-8591 (Fax)

Vinayak Ayurveda Center

2509 Virginia, NE
Albuquerque, NM 87110
(505) 296-6522
(505) 298-2932 (Fax)

Sources of Supply:

The following companies have an extensive selection of useful products and a long track-record of fulfillment. They have natural body care, aromatherapy, flower essences, crystals and tumbled stones, homeopathy, herbal products, vitamins and supplements, videos, books, audio tapes, candles, incense and bulk herbs, teas, massage tools and products and numerous alternative health items across a wide range of categories.

WHOLESALE:

Wholesale suppliers sell to stores and practitioners, not to individual consumers buying for their own personal use. Individual consumers should contact the RETAIL supplier listed below. Wholesale accounts should contact with business name, resale number or practitioner license in order to obtain a wholesale catalog and set up an account.

Lotus Light Enterprises, Inc.

P O Box 1008 ET
Silver Lake, WI 53170 USA
414 889 8501 (phone) 414 889 8591 (fax) 800 548 3824 (toll free order line)

RETAIL:

Retail suppliers provide products by mail order direct to consumers for their personal use. Stores or practitioners should contact the wholesale supplier listed above.

Internatural

33719 116th Street ET
Twin Lakes, WI 53181 USA
800 643 4221 (toll free order line) 414 889 8581 office phone
WEB SITE: www.internatural.com

Web site includes an extensive annotated catalog of more than 7000 products that can be ordered "on line" for your convenience 24 hours a day, 7 days a week.

INDEX

A

Agni, 26

Agnis, 86

Anatomy, Subtle, 30

Astrology, Vedic, 57

Attributes, 14

Ayurveda
- Ancient, 1, 3, 14, 57
- Rediscovered, 3
- Confirmation of, 71
- Modern, 1, 58

B

Body Seven Types, 11
- *See also* Srotas

Brahmana, Sakunteya, 72

Brihana
- *See* Therapy, Nourishing

C

Caste System, 187

Charaka, 58

Chinese Meridians, 75

Constitution, 12
- and Doshas, 81
- Determining, 16
- Seven Possible, 13
- Type, 59

Creative Play, 193

Curative Measures, 50

D

Dharma, 186

Dhatus, 22, 84

Direction, 36

Disease
- and the Planets, 75
- Eighth Category, 123, 149
- Etiology of, 33
- Symptomatology of, 41
- Tendencies, 59
- Three Pathways of, 46

Disease of All Types, 121
- Miscellaneous Symptoms, 123
- Seasonal, 122
- Time of Day, 122

Disease of Coldness, 65, 99, 132
- Aromatherapy, 134
- Blood Tissue, 100

Color and Gem Therapy, 134
Dietetics, 132
Endocrine System, 101
Eyes, 100
Face, 100
Feces, 99
Hatha Yoga, 133
Herbology, 132
Homeopathy, 132
Marma-Point and Acupuncture, 133
Massage, 133
Miscellaneous Symptoms, 102
Panchakarma, 132
Pericardium Meridian, 101
Pulse, 99
Skin, 100
Sound Therapy, 134
Tongue, 100
Triple-warmer Meridian, 101
Urine, 99
Voice, 100

Disease of Dryness, 69, 111, 142
Aromatherapy, 144
Color and Gem Therapy, 144
Dietetics, 142
Eyes, 112
Face, 112
Feces, 111
Hatha Yoga, 144
Herbology, 143
Homeopathy, 143
Marma-Point and Acupuncture, 144
Massage, 144
Miscellaneous Symptoms, 112
Muscle Tissue, 112
Panchakarma, 143
Pulse, 111
Skin, 111
Sound Therapy, 144
Spleen Meridian, 112
Stomach Meridian, 112
Tongue, 111
Urine, 111
Voice, 111

Disease of Heat, 67, 94, 127
Aromatherapy, 130
Bone Tissue, 95
Color and Gem Therapy, 130
Dietetics, 127
Endocrine System, 96
Eyes, 95
Face, 95
Feces, 94
Hatha Yoga, 129
Heart, 95
Herbology, 128
Homeopathy, 128
Marma-Point and Acupuncture, 130
Massage, 130
Miscellaneous Symptoms, 96
Panchakarma, 129
Pulse, 94
Skin, 94
Small Intestine Meridian, 95
Sound Therapy, 131
Tongue, 95

Urine, 94
Voice, 95
Disease of Heaviness, 62, 108, 138
Adipose Tissue, 109
Aromatherapy, 141
Color and Gem Therapy, 141
Conception Vessel, 109
Dietetics, 138
Endocrine System, 109
Eyes, 108
Face, 109
Feces, 108
Hatha Yoga, 140
Herbology, 139
Homeopathy, 140
Liver Meridian, 109
Marma-Point and Acupuncture, 140
Massage, 140
Miscellaneous Symptoms, 109
Panchakarma, 140
Pulse, 108
Skin, 108
Sound Therapy, 141
Tongue, 108
Urine, 108
Voice, 108
Disease of Lightness, 68, 103, 135
Aromatherapy, 137
Bone Marrow Tissue, 105
Color and Gem Therapy, 137
Dietetics, 135
Endocrine System, 105
Eyes, 105
Face, 105
Feces, 104
Gallbladder Meridian, 105
Governer Vessel, 105
Hatha Yoga, 137
Herbology, 136
Homeopathy, 136
Marma-Point and Acupuncture, 137
Massage, 137
Miscellaneous Symptoms, 106
Panchakarma, 136
Pulse, 103
Skin, 104
Sound Therapy, 138
Tongue, 104
Urine, 104
Voice, 104
Disease of Mixed Type, 70, 117, 148
Endocrine System, 119
Eyes, 118
Face, 118
Feces, 118
Large Intestine Meridian, 119
Lung Meridian, 119
Lymph Tissue, 118
Miscellaneous Symptoms, 119
Pulse, 118
Skin, 118
Tongue, 118
Urine, 118
Voice, 118

Disease of Oiliness, 63, 114, 145
Aromatherapy, 147
Bladder Meridian, 115
Color and Gem Therapy, 147
Dietetics, 145
Endocrine System, 116
Eyes, 115
Face, 115
Hatha Yoga, 147
Herbology, 146
Homeopathy, 146
Kidney Meridian, 116
Marma-Point Therapy, 147
Massage, 147
Miscellaneous Symptoms, 116
Panchakarma, 146
Pulse, 114
Reproductive Tissue, 115
Skin, 115
Sound Therapy, 147
Stool, 114
Tongue, 115
Urine, 114
Voice, 115
Doshas, 12
and Constitution, 81
Present Balance, 82
See also Vata, Pitta and Kapha

E
Eight Fields of Living, 5, 163
Endocrine System, 88
Etiology, 33

G
Geomancy, 177

H
Holistic Living, 163
Hormonal System, 76
Humour, 21
See also Dosha

K
Kapha, 12
Attributes of, 15
Five Forms of,
Avalambaka, 20
Bodhaka, 20
Kledaka, 20
Sleshaka, 20
Tarpaka, 20

L
Langhana
See Therapy, Lightening

M
Malas, 25, 85
Maudgalya, Purnaksa, 72
Mental Health, 176
Two Aspects of, 178
Mind, 37

O
Ojas, 30
Organs
of Action, 35
of Cognition, 34

P

Parasara, Maharishi, 60
Pathogenesis, 45
Physical Health, 165
Physiology, 30
Pitta, 12
  Attributes of, 15
  Five Forms of,
    Alochaka, 19
    Bhrajaka, 19
    Pachaka, 19
    Ranjaka, 19
    Sadhaka, 19
Planets
  and Disease, 75
  Jupiter, 60
  Mars, 60
  Mercury, 60
  Moon, 60
    North Node, 61
    South Node, 61
  Saturn, 61
  Sun, 60
  Venus, 61
Practitioner Guidelines, 154
Prakruti, 82
  See also Constitution
Prana, 17, 30
Prevention, 169
Preventive Measures, 49
Principles, Four Essential, 27
Professional Life, 189

R

Rasayana, 166
Regimen
  Daily, 170
  Food, 173
  Night, 174
  Seasonal, 175
Rejuvenation Therapy, 166
Relationships, 191
Rukshana
  See Therapy, Drying

S

Seasons, 122
Snehana
  See Therapy, Oleation
Soul, 38
Spirit, Eight Approaches to, 180
Spiritual Life, 179
Srotas, 27, 86
Stambana
  See Therapy, Astringent
Stress Management, 176
Suppression of Natural Urges, 175
Sushruta, 58
Swedana
  See Therapy, Fomentation

T

Taste
  Astringent, 69
  Bitter, 68
  Mixed, 70
  Pungent, 67
  Salty, 65
  Science of, 52

Science of the Seven, 11
Sour, 63
Sweet, 62
Tejas, 30
Therapeutics
Seven Basic, 11
Six-fold, 53
Therapy
Astringent, 54
Drying, 54
Fomentation, 54
Lightening, 53
Nourishing, 54
Oleation, 54
Time, 36, 122
Tissue
Functions, 23
Seven Elements, 11
See also Dhatus

V

Varyovida, 71
Vata, 12
Attributes of, 15
Five Forms of,
Apana, 18
Prana, 17
Samana, 17
Udana, 17
Vyana, 18
Vikruti, 82

W

Waste Products
See Malas
Wealth, 183